Costume & Civilization:

Louis XIV & Versailles

Costume & Civilization:

Louis XIV & Versailles

Diana de Marly

HM

Holmes & Meier
New York

First published in the United States of America 1987 by
Holmes & Meier Publishers, Inc.
30 Irving Place
New York, NY 10003

© Diana de Marly 1987

ISBN 0–8419–1148–7

Printed in Great Britain

Library of Congress Cataloging-in-Publication Data

De Marly, Diana.
    Louis XIV & Versailles.

    (Costume & civilization)
    Bibliography: p.
    Includes index.
    1. Costume–France–History–17th century.
2. Costume–France–History–18th century.   3. Louis
XIV, King of France, 1638-1715–Clothing.   I. Title.
II. Series.
GT857.D4   1987   391'.00944   87–25091
ISBN 0–8419–1148–7

Contents

Acknowledgements

Black and white photographs: Reproduced by Gracious Permission of Her Majesty Queen Elizabeth II, 2, 17, 24, 69. Amsterdam, the Rijksmuseum 3, 25; Berlin, Kunstbibliothek, Charlottenburg 33; Brussels, copyright ACL Institut Royal du Patrimoine Artistique 21, 32; Budapest, Hungarian National Museum 57; Cambridge, Fitzwilliam Museum 1, St John's College 79; Dijon, Musée des Beaux Arts 8; Grenoble, Musée des Beaux Arts 15; Honfleur, Musée du Vieux Honfleur 44, 45; London, the British Library 18, 23, 28, 29, National Gallery 78, National Portrait Gallery 49, Tate Gallery 36, Victoria and Albert Museum 51, 52, 55, 58, 61, 62, 63, 64, 66; Madrid, Museo del Prado 30; Marseilles, Musée des Beaux Arts 13, 34; Munich, Stadtmuseum von Parish collection 27, 37, 56, 65, 68, 71, 75, 76, 77; Duke of Northumberland 48; Oxford, the Ashmolean Museum 70; Paris, Bibliothèque Nationale 40, 41, 59, Giraudon 5, 6, 26, 35, Documentation Photographique de la Réunion des Musées Nationaux 4, 9, 10, 12, 14, 16, 19, 20, 22, 31, 34, 38, 39, 67, 72, 73; Saintes, Musée des Beaux Arts 80; Stockholm University Art Collection 11; Toledo Museum of Art, Ohio 74; Vienna, Kunsthistorisches Museum 7.

Colour photographs: London, the Wallace Collection 6; Madrid, Museo del Prado 4; Paris, Documentation Photographique de la Réunion des Musées Nationaux 1, 2, 3, 5, 7, 8.

The author is grateful to Professor Emeritus Ragnhild Hatton for discussing Louis XIV, to Dr Christian Michel of the Fondation Thiers for his paper 'Aspects de Propagande sous Louis XIV', to Madeleine Delpierre of the Musée de la Mode et du Costume, Paris, for her help over justaucorps, and to Stella Mary Newton for taking the photographs at Honfleur.

Chronology

1589 Henri IV first Bourbon king of France.

1598 Henri IV's Edict of Nantes gives freedom of worship to Protestant Reformed Church.

1601 Birth of Louis XIII, future father of Louis XIV.

1610 Henri IV assassinated. Queen mother Marie de' Medici Regent.

1615 Double marriage of French and Spanish dynasties.

1624 Cardinal Richelieu chief minister.

1638 Birth of Louis XIV on 5 September. Birth of his cousin and future wife the Infanta Maria Teresia of Spain on 20 September.

1640 Birth of brother Philippe, created Duc d'Orléans in 1660.

1642 Deaths of Cardinal Richelieu and Marie de' Medici. Cardinal Mazarin chief minister.

1643 Death of Louis XIII. Queen mother Anna Maria Mauritia Regent.

1648–59 War against Spain.

1648–53 The Fronde civil war in France.

1654 Coronation of Louis XIV at Rheims.

1659 Peace with Spain.

1660 9 June: marriage of Louis XIV to the Infanta Maria Teresia.

1661 9 March: death of Cardinal Mazarin. Louis XIV absolute monarch.
Marriage of Philippe Duc d'Orléans to Henriette Anne of England.
Louise de La Vallière becomes king's first mistress in July.
1 November: birth of son, Monseigneur Louis le Grand Dauphin.
Work starts on expanding Versailles.

1664–5 Great fêtes in the park at Versailles.

1666 Death of queen mother Anna Maria Mauritia.

1667 Gobelins re-established as a royal manufactory to supply Versailles.
Tariffs against Dutch and English goods.
Marquise de Montespan ousts La Vallière as principal mistress.

1667–8 War of Devolution. Louis XIV invades Spanish Netherlands and Franche Comté.

1670 Dutch boycott French goods. Secret Treaty of Dover between France and England.
Death of Henriette Anne Duchesse d'Orléans.

1671 Town of Versailles begun.
Philippe Duc d'Orléans married again to Elisabeth Charlotte of the Rhineland Palatinate.

1672–9   Louis XIV wars against the Dutch under William III of Orange.

1679   Marly-le-Roi begun as informal residence.

1680   Marriage of Monseigneur le Grand Dauphin to Victoire of Bavaria.

1682   Court and government moved to Versailles.

       Birth of first grandson Louis Duc de Bourgogne.

1683   Death of Queen Maria Teresia.

       Louis XIV's morganatic marriage to Marquise de Maintenon (precise date uncertain).

1683–6   War against Spain and Genoa.

1685   Revocation of Edict of Nantes. Huge eflux of Protestants from France.

1688–97   League of Augsburg formed to fight Louis XIV after he invaded the Rhineland Palatinate.

       Catholic James II deposed from British throne and replaced by his Protestant daughter Mary II and her cousin and husband William III of Orange. James takes refuge with Louis XIV.

1689   Britain's new monarchs ban French goods.

1693   Famine in France.

1696   Marriage arranged between Louis XIV's grandson Louis Duc de Bourgogne and Philippe's granddaughter Marie Adelaide of Savoy.

1697   Peace of Ryswick. Louis has to surrender most of his conquests.

1700   Carlos II of Spain bequeaths Spanish Empire to Louis XIV's second grandson Philippe Duc d'Anjou.

1701   William III settles Protestant succession in Britain: his cousin Princess Anne, then his mother's cousin Electress Sophia of Hanover and her son George.

1701   Death of Philippe Duc d'Orléans.

1702–14   Wars of the Spanish Succession.

1704   13 August: Marlborough defeats French at Blenheim.

1706   23 May: Marlborough defeats French at Ramillies.

1708   11 July: Marlborough and Prince Eugene defeat French at Oudenarde.

1708–9   Bitter winters cause poor harvests in France.

1709   Marlborough defeats French at Malplaquet.

1711   Louis XIV reduces tariffs against English, Danish and Norwegian goods.

       14 April: death of the heir Monseigneur Louis le Grand Dauphin.

1712   Deaths of Marie Adelaide Duchesse de Bourgogne, of grandson Louis Duc de Bourgogne and their son the Duc de Bretagne. Their other son survives to be Louis XV.

1713   Treaty of Utrecht. Louis XIV has to recognize Protestant succession in Britain. He yields Nova Scotia and Newfoundland to Britain. Spain yields Gibraltar and Minorca to Britain for naval bases.

1714   Death of third grandson the Duc de Berry after a riding accident.

       Louis XIV changes his will to include his bastards as princes of the blood.

       Deaths of Electress Sophia and Queen Anne mean that George of Hanover becomes King of Great Britain.

1715   1 September: death of Louis XIV. His nephew Philippe Duc d'Orléans is Regent for infant Louis XV. He moves court and government from Versailles back to Paris. Louis XIV's will is overturned and his bastards ousted.

1722   8 December: death of Regent's mother Elisabeth Charlotte Dowager Duchesse d'Orléans.

Introduction

'It is a miracle' declared the chief minister Cardinal Richelieu. 'He is the answer to all my prayers at long last!' cried the Queen Anna Maria Mauritia of the Spanish branch of the Hapsburg House of Austria. 'He is Louis the God Given, Louis le Dieudonné' said King Louis XIII of France. The birth of a son and heir at 11 a.m. on 5 September 1638 at the Château de St

1 Abraham Bosse, 'La Joye de la France', 1638.
The birth of Louis XIV on 5 September 1638 was seen as a miracle by many, for his parents had been married in 1615. The baby was tightly swaddled like any other child but was given a royal cloak and a crown. It was the end of the Cavalier style in fashion, as civil wars soon broke out in France and Britain, and were already raging in Germany. (*Fitzwilliam Museum, Cambridge*)

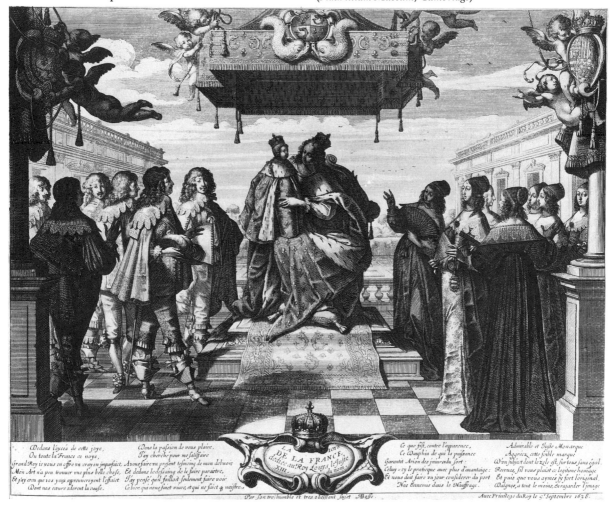

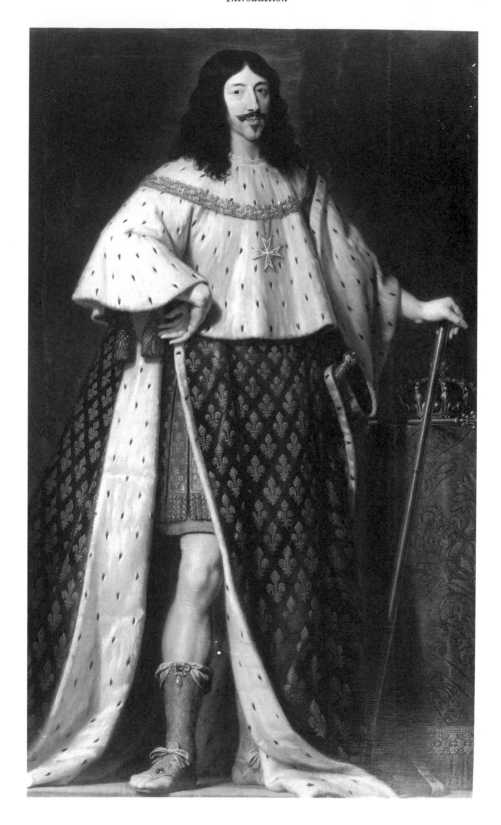

Germain to the king and queen after 23 years of marriage did indeed seem a miracle to many at the time. The king donated his crown to the Virgin Mary, and the queen built the convent of Val de Grâce in gratitude. Universal rejoicing was ordered across the country, although two branches of the royal family were not so pleased. The king's brother Gaston Duc d'Orléans had been his heir for the last 28 years, ever since the assassination of their father Henri IV in 1610, so he did not welcome his nephew's arrival. Gaston, however, had only daughters himself, and the French Salic law did not allow females to inherit the throne, so the heirs after Gaston were the males of the Bourbon princes de Condé. Their annoyance manifested itself in armed revolt ten years later. A second son, Philippe, followed on 22 September 1640.

Why Louis XIII should have taken so long to sire children has puzzled many historians ever since. Various explanations have been offered – that he disliked women because of his bossy mother Marie de' Medici who had been Regent during his minority. His health was often poor, although he loved hunting and dancing so he was not completely devoid of energy. Another explanation may be that Louis XIII's father Henri IV had been such a famous lover, whose bastards were frequenting the court for years to come, that his son possibly had a complex about equalling his reputation. This did not worry Louis XIII's son however, for the future Louis XIV would seek to outnumber his grandfather in the number of his illegitimate children. The site Louis XIV was to select for his intrigues, well away from the eyes of *maman* in the Louvre, was the hunting lodge that Louis XIII built at Versailles between 1624 and 1632. It had little room for guests, to keep his wife and mother away, and the marshy forest teemed with wolves, foxes and deer, which delighted young Louis when he first went there as a boy.

The Bourbon Dynasty was very new. Henri IV began as Henri of Navarre, a Protestant king, but inherited the French throne in 1589 from the last Valois, his father-in-law, and became a Catholic as it was a Catholic kingdom which had seen several massacres of the Protestants shortly before then. Henri IV protected the reformed Church by his Edict of Nantes in 1598 which gave Protestants freedom of worship and the right to garrison four towns. The Catholic Church resolved to destroy this edict as soon as it got the chance and the appointment of Cardinal Richelieu as chief minister in 1624 saw the start: he cancelled the clause allowing Protestant garrisons and starved La Rochelle into submission in 1628 in defiance of her rights by treaty and law. This set the pattern which Louis XIV was to follow. Richelieu initiated a policy which was happy with contradictions. The Hapsburgs were the most powerful dynasty in Europe, and their lands enclosed France from the Spanish Netherlands in the north, down through the Holy Roman Empire to Italy and Austria , and so to Spain in the south, with her overseas empire in the Americas. The Hapsburgs were fellow Catholics, but Richelieu gladly encouraged Protestants in their realms to undermine Hapsburg power, and actually joined the Thirty Years War on the Protestant side. Inside France, however, the opposite policy was pursued of persecuting Protestants with the intention of extinguishing the reformed Church completely. When Richelieu died in 1642 his policy was continued by the new chief minister, the Italian Cardinal Mazarin, who passed it on to Louis XIV when Louis XIII made the cardinal responsible for his heir's education. The dynasty which began with a change of faith had to be more Catholic than the Pope, at home.

The root of French policy was to detach Spain from the Hapsburgs. This started in 1615 with the double marriage of the teenagers Louis XIII of France to the Infanta Anna Maria Mauritia of Spain, and of his sister Princess Elizabeth of France to the Infante Philip Prince of Asturias, who was Anna's brother, and became King Philip IV in 1621. This close mixing of the two families continued with two other royal marriages that century and in 1700 reached its culmination when Carlos II bequeathed Spain to France. A serious attempt was also made all the century to detach Britain from the Protestant fold, beginning with the marriage of Louis XIII's sister Henriette Marie to Charles I of England and Scotland. This did lead in 1685 to the occupation of the British throne by an open Roman Catholic, James II, but within three years he had been ousted, and replaced by his Protestant daughter Mary II and her

---

2 Philippe de Champaigne, 'Louis XIII'.
The father of Louis XIV was considered a mystery by many, and died when his heir was five. Underneath his royal mantle he wears Roman armour which Cosimo III had revived at his court in Florence in the 1550s as the ideal imperial image for monarchy. This concept was brought to France by the Medici princesses such as Louis XIII's mother Marie de' Medici, and handed down to Louis XIV for his official images. (*Reproduced by Gracious Permission of Her Majesty the Queen*)

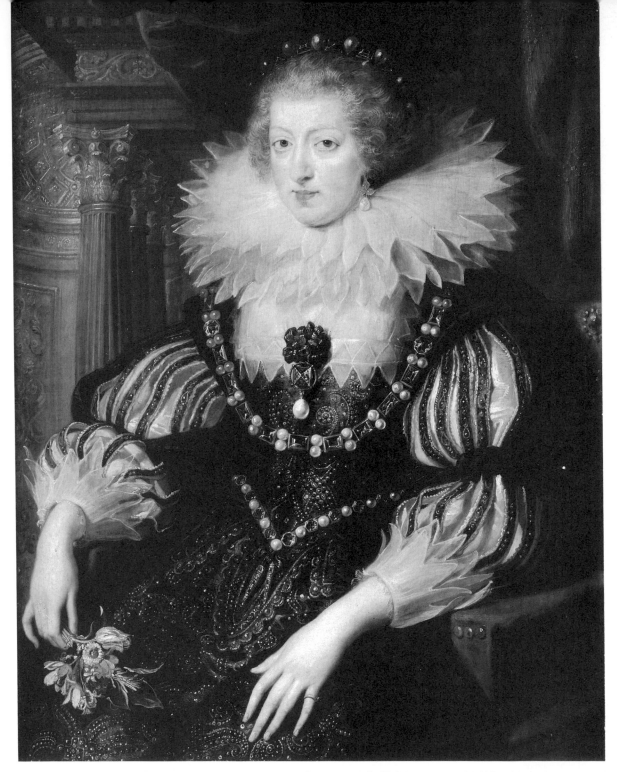

3 Peter Paul Rubens, 'Anna Maria Mauritia Queen of France', *c.* 1635.

The mother of Louis XIV had experienced miscarriages in 1618 and 1630, but had to wait for 23 years of marriage to produce a successful pregnancy. A Spaniard by birth of the Hapsburg dynasty, she had been stripped of Spanish styles at the moment of marriage. She here wears the height of French fashion with puffed, slashed sleeves, her ruff and cuffs cut like petals, and the dress covered with seed-pearl embroidery. Royalty was required to look magnificent even when feeling miserable. (*Rijksmuseum Amsterdam*)

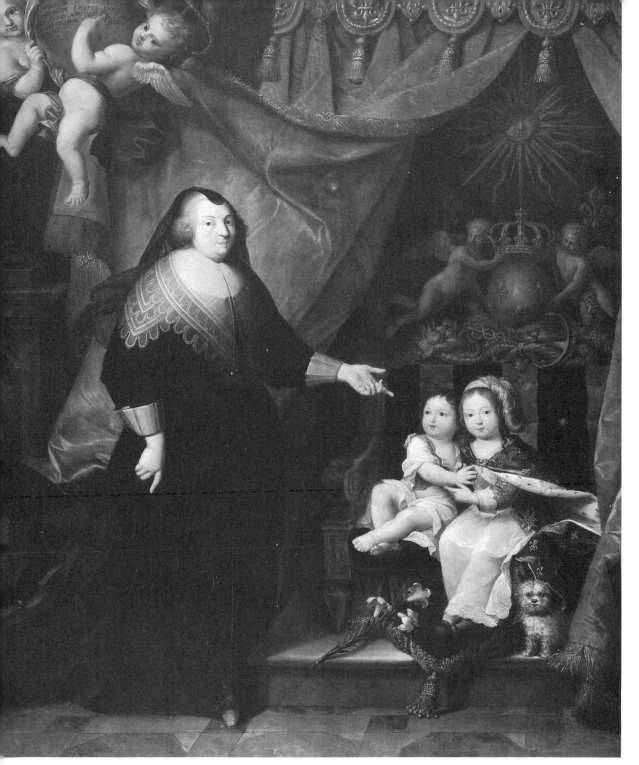

4 French School, 'Madame de Lansac with the Children of France', 1641.

A second son, Philippe, was born in 1640, and is here portrayed at one, with Louis XIV now three. The infant prince wears the usual petticoats and apron of baby boys but with the Order of the Saint Esprit, a royal cloak lined with ermine, and a cap with an ostrich plume to indicate status. The boys are seen with their widowed governess. They were probably painted by the court artist Justus van Egmont, but the remainder of the picture is by lesser hands. Note the solar image behind the throne. It was chosen for Louis by his parents. (*Versailles, cliché des Musées Nationaux*)

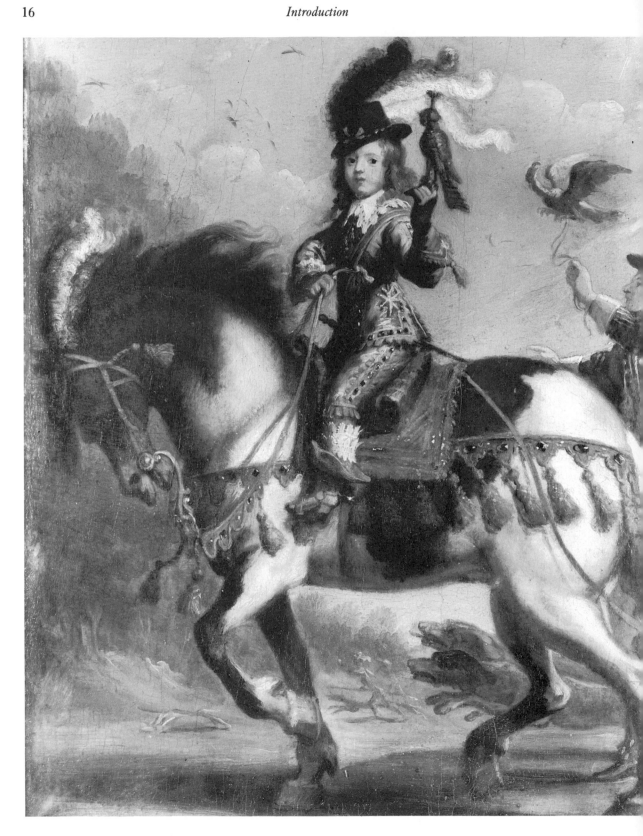

Dutch husband William of Orange, and the British counter-attack seriously undermined French successes. There were also regular marriages with Savoy, from Louis XIII's sister Chrétienne to the Duke Victor Amadeus I and onwards, with the ultimate intention of incorporating the duchy into France. In 1635 Richelieu occupied the duchy of Lorraine. The expansion of France was duly undertaken by Louis XIV in continuance of Richelieu's example, into the territories belonging mainly to the Hapsburgs.

The death of Richelieu in 1642 was followed that same year by the death of Louis XIV's grandmother Marie de' Medici, and in April 1643 by the death of his father Louis XIII before his heir was five years old. There had to be another regency, with his mother and Cardinal Mazarin running the kingdom on young Louis's behalf. In fact the cardinal was so devoted to the Queen Regent that the Dutch printed a pamphlet claiming that he was Louis XIV's father, stating 'how closely he [Louis XIV] ressembles his Eminence – the same haughty glance, the same uncontrolled passion for pompous buildings, luxurious dress and retinues, the same deference and devotion to the queen mother'.[1] Certainly the cardinal influenced his young charge greatly in his tastes in art and architecture, and in the aims of kingship. His mother, though a Hapsburg, had been born in Spain and had arrived in France in full Spanish attire with a closed ruff, a farthingale and long hanging sleeves, and used to sit on cushions on the floor in the Moorish tradition. She had been given a more French look with falling ruffs and less voluminous skirts, but she still spoke with a Spanish accent and was deeply devout. The young king had to wait on his mother the Regent at her levée, and hand her her chemise as she dressed for mass in a long black mourning cloak. The court wore deep mourning for the first year, with Louis in violet and the court in black. Richelieu had not allowed the queen to keep any Spanish ladies as companions but the moment he died she sent for Françoise de Motteville who had a Spanish mother, and appointed

her a woman-in-waiting. She was not noble enough to be a lady-in-waiting, but she spoke Spanish, and she wrote a valuable memoir of the reign. Thus there was a strong Spanish flavour of strict religious observance which influenced Louis XIV for the remainder of his life, for he always performed the religious duties with solemnity and regularity, even if he cared less for the actual principles of the Church. Needless to say, the Queen Regent adored her elder son. After 23 years of humiliation and shame, when she had been afraid of being sent back to Spain in disgrace for not producing any children, and had thought of asking her father Philip III for another post as viceroy for the Spanish Netherlands, the arrival of young Louis le Dieudonné had indeed seemed like a miracle, the reward for 23 years of prayer.

Louis XIV was breeched and taken out of baby petticoats in time for the first big international event of his reign, the proxy marriage in Paris of Princess Louisa Maria Gonzaga to King Ladislas IV of Poland in 1645; the Poles had asked the French court to select a suitable princess. The party of Poles arrived looking very Turkish with their shaved heads with only one tuft of hair remaining, and the officers wore Turkish jackets and caftans with wide sleeves much enriched with jewels. The Polish nobles wore heavy brocade caftans with diamond buttons. Some of their horses were painted red. Madame de Motteville was surprised at the absence of linen and thought the Poles did not wear it but preferred furs for lining clothes and in place of sheets. The bride was attired all in white and silver, the usual choice for royal weddings in the seventeenth century, with a white bodice and a cloth of silver petticoat to harmonize with the Polish royal mantle of white velvet embroidered in gold. How the crown should sit upon her fashionable coiffure posed a problem, so it was the hairdresser Mme de Senécé who decided exactly how it should be worn. Another colourful event was a visit from Queen Christina of Sweden in September 1646, with her staff all in yellow and black decorated with silver lace.

The young king was dressed in colourful ways once mourning was over. In 1647 he danced in a comedy before Cardinal Mazarin and the Queen Regent dressed in doublet and kneebreeches of black satin heavily embroidered with silver and gold, and trimmed with cherry-coloured ribbons and cherry plumes on his hat. Heavy embroidery was the height of fashion, and some of the best examples survive in the Royal Armoury in Stockholm which has several suits belonging to King Carl X. His coronation suit for

---

5 Jean de Saint Igny, 'Louis XIV Hawking'.
Louis XIV first saw his father's hunting lodge at Versailles when Louis XIII took him hunting. After his father's death Louis continued to hunt there and grew very attached to the freedom it gave. He is here about six or seven, king in name, although his mother was the Regent. He has been breeched into an adult-typed suit with the narrower sleeves and smaller collars of the 1640s. His hawksman wears a braided livery. (*Musée Condé, Chantilly; photograph Giraudon*)

the ceremony in Upsala Cathedral on 6 June 1654 is so smothered with embroidery that the fabric is invisible. The embroidery was padded and raised, and became increasingly heavy as the century advanced. Louis XIV liked jewels to be incorporated in the pattern and ultimately the weight was to be self-defeating. In 1651 when Louis XIV came of age, and Mazarin started taking him to meetings of the council of state, there was a triumphant parade through Paris with Louis in a suit smothered in gold embroidery, while his horse's caparison was embroidered with fleur de lys and the crosses of the Holy Ghost, the order of the Saint Esprit. He was preceded by the Grand Equerry of France the Comte d'Harcourt in doublet and hose of gold and silver cloth, his horse covered with crimson velvet embroidered with gold. There were six heralds in crimson velvet tabards embroidered with the fleur de lys in gold, with velvet caps and carrying the caduceus. Six royal trumpeters wore blue velvet. The Swiss Guard wore a historical uniform with a ruff, doublet and melon-shaped breeches of the style of about 1600, with black velvet caps, gold cords and plumes. The King's Troop of Light Horse had coats of gold and silver cloth and plain cloth, while their four trumpeters were in blue velvet laced with gold and silver. The Queen Regent's Troop was led by a lieutenant in a coat embroidered with gold and silver, and had four trumpeters in black velvet trimmed with silver lace.[2] All this royal display was essential for a serious challenge to the regency, and Cardinal Mazarin had broken out.

The revolt of the Fronde, the sling, began in 1648 when the Paris Parlement were influenced by the way the English Parliament had beaten their king. They were annoyed first by the Crown preparing to appoint a large number of new magistrates when the existing magistrates had paid a high price for their positions. Many posts in French administration were for sale, as were the titles of marquis and comte which belonged to an estate and could be purchased with it, like the lord-of-the-manor system in England. Dukes and princes were created by the monarch, however. Parlement demanded that the value of their posts be maintained and taxes on the poor be relieved. The Queen Regent did reduce court pay, but Parlement went on to demand tax cuts, the right to inspect the taxes and fines, and the right to inspect prison cases where a person had been arrested for over 24 hours. An old army officer, Broussel, spoke up for the heavily taxed people and the Regent unwisely had him arrested. The barricades went up and the Queen

Regent and her sons had to leave Paris in a hurry. Parlement banned and exiled Cardinal Mazarin, and banned all cardinals from becoming chief ministers.

The second stage of the Fronde developed when the other members of the royal family, notably Gaston Duc d'Orléans and the Prince de Condé, combined against Mazarin. They resented the centralization which had been going on since Henri IV and which threatened their feudal independence and they took up arms against the Mazarins party, that is the Queen Regent, the boy king Louis XIV, general Turenne, and the exiled cardinal. To tell the forces apart Condé's troops wore straw in their hats, and the Mazarins paper. Gaston's eldest daughter, Anne Marie Louise Duchesse de Montpensier, galloped off to Orléans in her Amazon habit of a man's coat and hat to secure the city for her father, and later fired the cannon of the Bastille upon the royal troops. She did say that Condé was the most slovenly dressed prince she knew, but for the revolt he smartened himself up and wore a coat with the party colour blue in a scarf across the front, German style. As a fashion note, Anne Marie Louise observed that it was the start of the winter season when people had to parade at the Tuileries in new clothes. Her own colours were red, white and black, and when the impoverished King Charles II was in exile in France he had worn her colours on his hat, swordknot, gloves and stockings as he tried to court Mademoiselle and her fortune, but she had no time for kings without a kingdom. The Fronde dragged on until 1653 when dissension among the Orléans party allowed the court to return to Paris from Saint Germain and Cardinal Mazarin was recalled.[3]

It all gave the young king a nasty shock – Paris mobs, barricades, untrustworthy uncles and cousins, a Parlement trying to grab more power. It was with great eagerness that he listened to the cardinal's advice: give the nobility privileges but no power, exclude the aristocracy from your counsels, choose

6 Philippe de Champaigne, *Cardinal Mazarin.*
Giulio Mazarini began as officer in the Pope's army, but entered the Church as a diplomat in 1630. Sent to France, he entered the service of Louis XIII in 1636 and was trained by Cardinal Richelieu to succeed him as chief minister. Louis XIII entrusted him with the education of his elder son, the heir Louis. Relations between the cardinal, the queen mother and the boy king were very close, but he was detested by other branches of the royal family who fought against him. He was created a cardinal in 1642. (*Musée Condé, Chantilly; photograph Giraudon*)

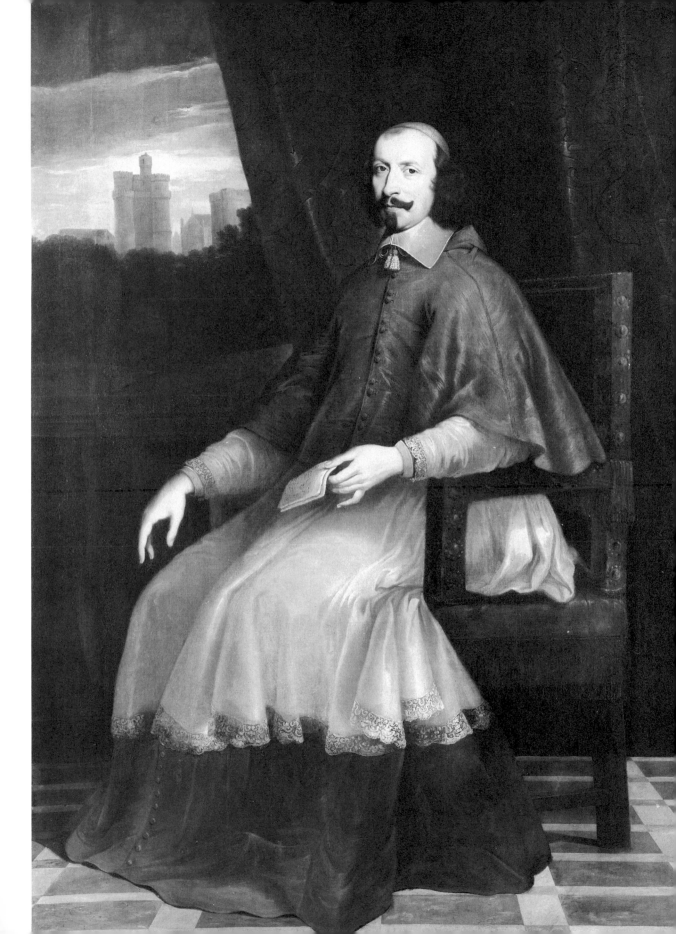

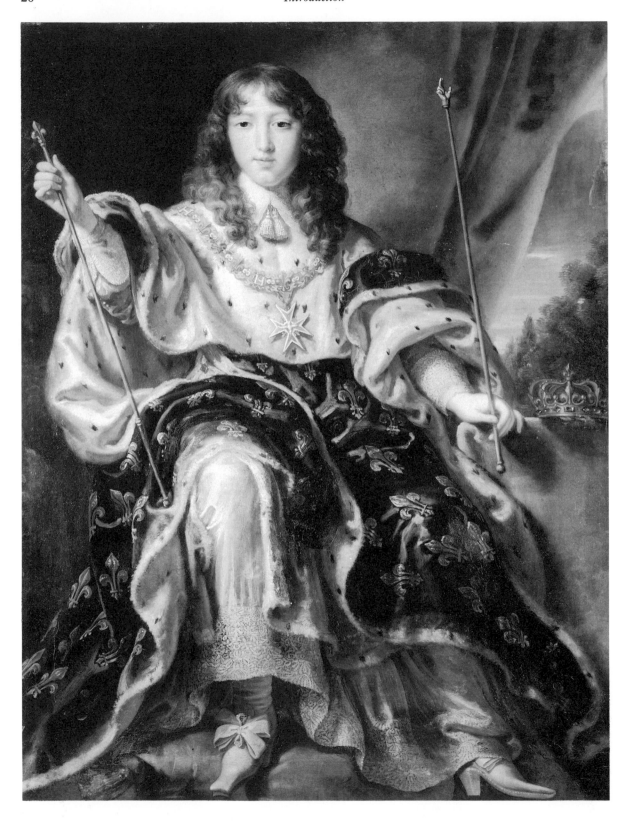

your ministers from among the bourgeoisie who will thus be in your debt, and always be your own chief minister when His Eminence has passed away. The Fronde having been defeated, the coronation could now proceed at Rheims on 7 June 1654, and Nicolas Sanctot, subsequently master of ceremonies at Versailles, described it. The king's brother Philippe, now 13, arrived in ducal attire with his train carried by his master of the wardrobe the Marquis de Viantes. All the dukes had vests of cloth of gold, mantles lined with ermine, and ducal crowns. The masters of the ceremonies wore a livery in the sixteenth-century style of cloth of silver doublets and black velvet trunkhose slashed, with pearl grey stockings, and black velvet mantles lined with cloth of silver and embroidered with silver, and black velvet toques with white ostrich plumes. The drummers, trumpeters and players of the hautbois were all in white taffeta, and the heralds were in white velvet with white silk stockings attached to their trunkhose, with the royal coat of arms across their chests.

Louis XIV, not yet 16, arrived with the Swiss Guards. He wore a tunic of violet satin under a nightgown robe of cloth of silver, and a black velvet toque garnished with white ostrich plumes and a double aigrette. At the altar the nightgown was removed and handed to the first valet of the chamber, Sieur de Niel. The toque was handed to Prince Eugene who transferred it to the first valet of the wardrobe, Sieur Moreau. The grand chamberlain placed the violet velvet shoes, embroidered with the fleur de lys in gold, upon the king's feet. Then came the anointing and the donning of the tunic, dalmatic and royal mantle of violet velvet embroidered with golden fleur de lys. Louis was handed the sceptre and the hand of justice, and the crowning followed, after which a Te Deum was sung.[4]

John Evelyn had seen the young king in 1651 riding from Parlement: 'The King himselfe like a young *Apollo* was in a sute so covered with rich embrodry that one could perceive nothing of the stuff under it, going almost the whole way with his hat in his hand saluting the Ladys & Acclamators.'[5] While it is often thought that Louis chose the god Apollo as his image, he was in fact being presented as such by the Queen Regent and Cardinal Mazarin in the court ballets where he danced as the deity. Such ballets were tradition and his father had danced in the Christmas ballet of 1625 when he had appeared as a Spanish guitar player with a cape of pink satin in the Spanish style. The bills for this ballet have been published by Danjou, along with the account of the royal perfumer Jehan Dufour for supplying Louis XIII with six sachets of roses for his bed and clothes. [6] This nicety the queen mother passed on to young Louis who became very particular about clean linen. The Venetian ambassador in 1652 had commented that 'Games, dances and comedies are the King's sole pursuits', but after his coronation Louis was sent off to spend his summers with the army, returning to the court for the winter season. In the meantime his cousin Gaston's daughter Anne Marie Louise Duchesse de Montpensier went off to the spa at Forges for the winter of 1656, and observed that morning costumes were of fur and cloth but after dinner, at midday, taffeta was obligatory. She attended the court masked ball in 1658 attired in cloth of gold and silver with a plumed hat, and said that all the men wore highly embroidered suits and silk stockings. France waged war against Spain from 1635 to 1659 and gained Rousillon and Cerdagne, so a peace treaty was now in order. Unfortunately young Louis XIV fell head over heels in love with Cardinal Mazarin's youngest niece, Marie Mancini. This did not accord with French foreign policy. Spain had to be detached from Austria, so Louis must marry his cousin the Spanish Infanta Maria Teresia, daughter of Philip IV and his aunt Elizabeth of France, now deceased. His mother delivered lectures on royal duties overriding personal feelings, and while Cardinal Mazarin found good husbands for all his nieces he told the king that they were not of the blood royal, and were thus unfit for his sacred role. Louis XIV gave in.

In the midst of the preparations uncle Gaston Duc d'Orléans died on 2 February 1660 and Anne Marie Louise put the household into black. However, curiosity overcame filial devotion, and she went to the Spanish border for the royal wedding. It was said that her part in the Fronde had cost her the post of royal bride, but the duchess was far too independent to have put up with Louis XIV and his future *affaires*. The title

7 Justus van Egmont, 'The Coronation Portrait of Louis XIV', 1654.
After the collapse of the Fronde Louis was crowned at Rheims on 7 June 1654, dressed in the tunic, dalmatic and royal mantle of blue strewn with the fleur de lys in gold. He carries the sceptre, and the hand of justice which was supposed to be his special concern. Justus van Egmont trained under Rubens alongside Van Dyck, and became a French court artist in the 1640s, and an elder of the Royal Academy of Painting and Sculpture in 1663.
(*Kunsthistorisches Museum, Vienna; photograph Alpenland*)

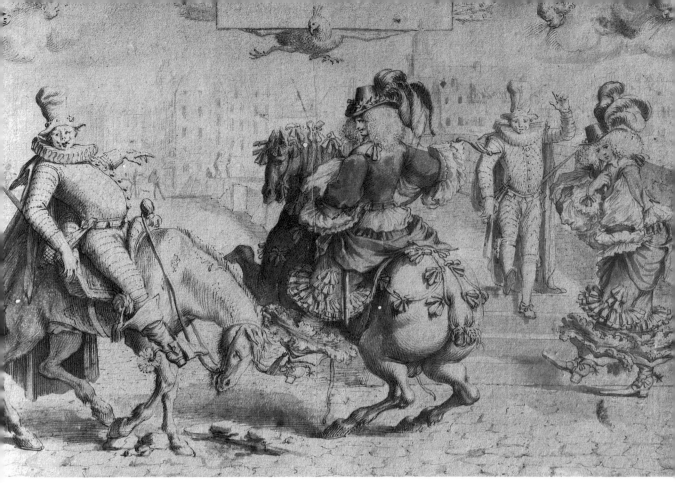

of Duc d'Orléans now passed to Louis XIV's brother Philippe who became styled Monsieur le Duc d'Orléans, as the title was the prerogative of the king's brother, so their cousin Anne could not inherit it. Anne was often called La Grande Mademoiselle as she was the biggest heiress and now the richest lady in France in her own right. She examined the Spanish Infanta who was dressed in a white satin farthingale embroidered with knots of silver lamé. The king of Spain was in a grey suit embroidered with silver.

The meeting of the two courts was the most famous costume clash of the century, for they operated completely different approaches. As France had been an enemy and a challenge to Hapsburg rule of Europe, Philip IV in 1623 had introduced his *Capitulos de Reformacion* and banned the French styles of huge lace collars, long hair, and clothes slashed and embroidered. In the Spanish empire all officials and courtiers had to wear a plain doublet and narrow kneebreeches, and the special golilla collar of plain white linen stiffened with shellac, instead of immoderate ruffs. The king had also tried to control farthingales but the queens were excepted and they continued to wear farthingales which were a Spanish

8 Louis Testelin, 'French Luxury Victorious over Spanish Pride', *c.* 1656.

The competition between French and Spanish fashions was intense and reflected the political enmity. By now Louis XIV was 18; he adopted French luxury and excess with enthusiasm and promoted it fully. The old idea of slashing was taken to a new extreme with the shirt bursting out of the sleeves and around the waist. Ribbon was worn all over from the hat to the knee, and bucket-top boots were the rage. The Spanish in contrast tried to maintain a conservative and dignified appearance, although not quite so antique as the millstone ruffs and peascod bellies the artist has mocked them with here. (*Musée des Beaux Arts, Dijon, cliché des Musées Nationaux*)

invention, and seem to be in keeping with the desire of Spanish men to isolate their women from other males. The Infanta Maria Teresia had been born in 1638, so she was almost the same age as Louis XIV, and she had been raised like a nun. The French court was going to prove a terrific shock, and she did not speak French. Thus her aunt and mother-in-law to be, Anne Maria Mauritia of Austria, queen mother and former Regent of France, was going to be her greatest ally and refuge, as she spoke Spanish, and had been an Infanta herself.

In contrast the French court loved embroidery, display, and frivolty. Louis XIV was 21 and he wanted to shine so that the whole world could see Apollo in his splendour. He wanted his clothes to be more and more fantastic and extremely lively, the opposite to Spanish sobriety. The trend all through the 1650s was for doublets to grow shorter, but Louis wore them shorter still. Kneebreeches had been tubular in the 1640s but then grew wider, which was all they could do after being narrow, and by 1658 the rhinegraves or petticoat breeches, had appeared. They were decorated with satin ribbons by the yard, indeed by the mile, for the French court sported them all over. The favourite colours were sky blue, yellow, and all the tones of red, scarlet, crimson, cherry and flame ('couleur de feu'). Louis XIV loved flame in particular, for it represented the flames of the sun of which Apollo was the god: the king should glow with flame-coloured satin ribbons and plumes, as he was King Sun on earth. Madame de Motteville opined that the younger generation had gone too far: 'I

thought the dress of the Frenchmen ridiculous with huge bow-knots of ribbon on their legs, and found much to say against their little doublets which covered neither their bodies nor their stomachs.' The ribbons were worn on the hats, on the sword handles, on canes, on the sleeve, round the waist, round the knees,

9 Charles Le Brun, 'The Meeting of Louis XIV with Philip IV of Spain on the Island of Pheasants', 1660.
The most famous costume clash of the century. On the right the Spanish, with the men in doublets and kneebreeches with golilla collars, their own hair, and flat shoes. The Infanta Maria Teresia wears a farthingale. The French sport long hair or periwigs, short doublets, petticoat breeches, masses of ribbon, and high-heeled shoes, with Monsieur Philippe the king's brother in the highest heels of all, which he was to make even higher next year. One courtier with his back to the spectator, shows the brand new combination of a coat with kneebreeches to form a new type of suit. Sleeves had become voluminous again. Behind Louis XIV are the queen mother and cardinal Mazarin. (*Tapestry in the French Embassy, Madrid; cliché des Musées Nationaux*)

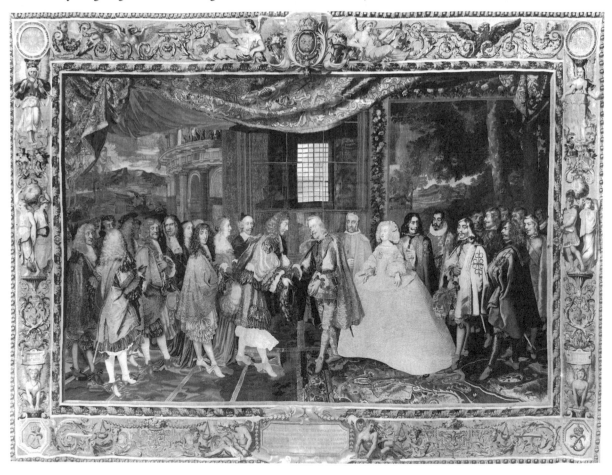

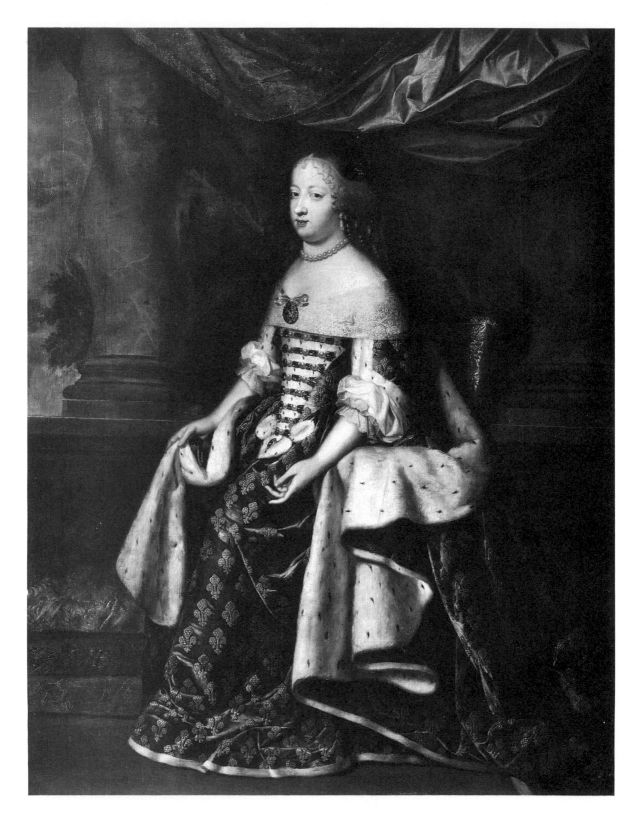

and on the shoes. A great bunch of ribbon was placed over the stomach as if to remind spectators that while the man was wearing petticoat breeches, he was a physical male underneath. It was an extreme style, but it is a tendency of youth to worship the excitement of extremism and Louis XIV was a young monarch. Madame de Motteville much preferred the Spanish style, but she was half Spanish: 'The grandees do not wear clothes so much embroidered as those of Frenchmen; but on their plain and simple stuffs they all had splendid jewels, which distinguished them from common people, and gave them a fine appearance. Their clothes had grace, although their breeches were too narrow, just as those of the Frenchmen looked deformed by their width.' It was a visual display of political fact, two competing courts promoting different fashions as they strove to defeat each other. The Spanish court style was compulsory in the Spanish empire, and in the Austrian empire, and several Catholic states in Germany adopted it too. No visitor to the courts of Vienna or Madrid could be received except in Spanish dress. The French, however, were striving very hard to promote their fashion and their culture. While this royal marriage between the two countries was a pledge of peace, it was a promise that Louis XIV and Mazarin had no intention of honouring.

None of the French liked the Infanta's clothes, with her monstrous farthingale, very dated hanging sleeves, the false hair in the wide style exposing her forehead, and thought the slashing on the sleeves to be in poor taste. For the first meeting with her husband-to-be the Infanta Maria Teresia wore a farthingale dress of white satin embroidered with birds, and with a border of the French royal fleur de lys. There was no kissing, for the King of Spain did not kiss people, and even the queen mother of France, his own sister whom he had not seen for 45 years, received the coolest salute. The Infanta, however, embraced her aunt warmly and placed herself under her protection.

For the final wedding ceremony on 9 June 1660

Louis XIV wore black, the most fashionable and respectable shade and a perfect ground for coloured ribbons, and the Infanta wore a white brocade embroidered with talc, as silver was banned by Spanish sumptuary law, with a royal mantle of purple velvet embroidered with fleur de lys. That very night, as soon as the new queen of France was in French hands, her Spanish clothes were stripped from her, in the same way as her mother-in-law's Spanish clothes had been taken from her in 1615. It was the Duchess de Navaille as lady of honour who threw out all the farthingales, and put the new queen into a blue dress covered with fleur de lys and trimmed with ermine. Louis XIV changed for the evening festivities into a suit of cloth of silver, in the French fashion. Not only was the queen's wardrobe translated entirely into French, so was her name, and Maria Teresia became Marie Thérèse. Her state entry into Paris was designed by the lesser royal artists the Beaubrun brothers, and she wore black embroidered with gold, silver and precious stones, which showed off her blond hair and blue eyes very well.[7] Louis XIV was also blond of a dark tone, with blue-black eyes and olive skin. His grandmother Marie de' Medici had been a true Rubens blonde and passed something of her looks on to Louis, but his brother Philippe was a total contrast, very dark and a head shorter than the king.

The first shock to the new queen was that her outer clothes were to be put on her by male tailors. She asked Louis XIV to change the system but he refused. Lacing the queen was the prerogative of her tailors and the valets of the wardrobe. As so many women at court were wearing low necklines why should the queen worry about who dressed her? The queen was obliged to accept the system but loathed it and insisted on donning her shift, petticoats and stockings unaided behind a screen.[8] A second shock was that Cardinal Mazarin put his financial expert Colbert in charge of the queen's income; he allowed her only a 1,000 crowns a month for minor pleasures, and cut her New Year's present to 10,000 crowns. The queen mother protested that Louis XIII had always given her 12,000 crowns, but Colbert believed in economies. Then there was the new queen's brother-in-law Monsieur Philippe. There were plenty of masked balls following the royal wedding, and Philippe appeared at one dressed as a woman with a blond wig and dress, and was delighted when a man dressed as a monk tried to court him. Anne Marie Louise was amused and allowed Philippe to appear with her as shepherdesses

---

10 Attributed to the Beaubruns, 'The Infanta Maria Teresia turned into Queen Marie Thérèse of France', 1660.

The Spanish farthingales were thrown away, the hair restyled into French ringlets, and the Infanta was translated into a French queen with the royal blue velvet strewn with gold fleur de lys. As yet there was no court dress as such, so she wore the fashionable style in royal fabrics. (*Versailles*)

in dresses of silver tissue, with rose-coloured piping, and black velvet aprons, roughly in the style of peasants on her estates at Bresanne but with fashionable collars and cuffs which were much wider than those worn by the peasantry. Their hats were in black velvet with red, white and black plumes, their bodices were laced with pearls and fastened with diamonds. The shepherds' crooks were of red lacquer decorated with silver. The new queen had never heard of homosexuality. That year Cardinal Mazarin told Anne Marie Louise that he and the queen mother were very worried about Monsieur's transdressing and wanted to stop it. They thought he ought to join the army but Philippe refused and clung to *maman*.

Several modern historians claim that his mother deliberately tried to turn Philippe into a homosexual by dressing him as a girl when he was young so he would not threaten his brother, as uncle Gaston had done. This is nonsense. All boys wore petticoats when they were babies. It was the normal thing to do right into this century. Boys were usually breeched between five and eight, although it might be delayed if they were sickly or else too small, like Philippe. Moreover the queen mother was deeply religious and was to be as horrified by Louis XIV's adultery as by Philippe's perversion. She did not want either son to be a sinner. As the king's brother, Philippe was protected from being hanged or burned for his offence, and his sexual preferences served as sensational publicity for the French court. *Les Pourtraicts de la Cour*, published at Cologne in 1667, said of Monsieur 'he is not, however, so Majestick as the King, mild, agreable, civil, and obliging, very complaisant to the Ladies, always gay and active, curious of rarieties, and nice in his Habits and Modes.' Louis XIV was much grander: 'He *Dances* admirably and though he wears sometimes a *disguise*, yet his Majestick Garb, and Ayre doth soon discover him.'[10]

Philippe might not be the sort of publicity Louis XIV wanted, but propaganda and publicity were the basis of his approach. The arts were nationalized, or should one say 'royalized', into a system of glorification of the king. The Paris Academy of Art, founded in 1648, was taken over as the Académie Royale de Peinture et de Sculpture in 1661. The Académie des Inscriptions et Belles Lettres was founded in 1663 with special responsibility for panegyrics and celebrations of the monarch, in 1669 the Académie Royale de Musique et de Danse was established to sing and dance to the king's glory, and in 1671 the Académie Royale d'Architecture was set up to build palatial magnificence to accommodate this sun god. The number of printers was reduced to make censorship easier, and nothing that did not praise the monarch could expect to appear in France (so criticism was published in Amsterdam).

On 1 November 1661 Queen Marie Thérèse presented Louis with a son, the Grand Dauphin Monseigneur Louis, although only he survived out of the total of six children the queen bore by 1672. In his *Instruction of the Dauphin* Louis XIV set down his ideas as received from Mazarin: the King of France is the equal of emperors! Ministers love to feel that they have a master. Never allow judicial associations like the Parlement of Paris to acquire any sovereignty. Corrupt the English court with bribes to undo the Protestant establishment. It is essential to maintain sovereign authority undivided. The English system (where his cousin Charles II had to answer to Parliament) 'is a perversion of the order of things to assign decisions to subjects and submission to the sovereign'. The king was responsible to God alone. He was Absolute. Cardinal Mazarin died on 9 March 1661, and Louis XIV dutifully announced that he would be his own chief minister, which people did not believe. He was too fond of hunting and dancing for government committees to interest him long, but he stuck to it. Next day, 10 March, Louis XIV excluded from his council the queen mother and former Regent, his brother who was a shocking gossip, and the marshalls Prince Condé and Turenne. He relied on the team Mazarin had established: Nicolas Fouquet Marquis de Belle-Ile, Comte de Melun et de Vaux the Superintendent of Finances since 1653, Jean Baptiste Colbert the cardinal's general factotum since the 1640s, Michel le Tellier as secretary of state, and Hugues de Lionne for war. The aristocracy might sneer, but these families were not nobodies and had been climbing up the society tree for generations.[11] Absolute rule began.

ONE

The French Impact 1660–1680

Europe was interested to see how France's young king would cope on his own. The court was still small and itinerant in the 1660s in the medieval tradition, moving around its seats from the Louvre, to Chambord, to Fontainebleau, to Saint Germain, to Compiègne, and to Versailles lodge for the hunting. Louis XIV's personal reign opened with a number of scandals. Firstly, there was high-heeled shoes for men. Following his marriage to his cousin Princess Henriette Anne of England in 1661, Monsieur Philippe the king's brother said that he now had a claim to the English throne after his wife's brother Charles II and James Duke of York, and put all his servants into English royal scarlet liveries. Henriette Anne giggled at the whole idea. She said Monsieur was so short and so ridiculous in the way he dressed with scents, lace and diamonds that the English would laugh him off the throne. Much stung by this reference to his lack of height Monsieur sent for his shoemaker Lambertin and told him to put an extra two inches into the heels of his shoes. Henriette Anne told Louis XIV what his brother was up to, so when Monsieur swaggered into court wearing his high heels he was astounded to see the king still towering above him because he had increased his heels too. Consternation! How could he? But nobody was allowed to outshine the king. No doubt Monsieur complained mightily to the queen mother, but Louis XIV took to high heels and kept them the fashion at court right up to 1715.[1]

Another scandal seemed imminent when Louis XIV started flirting with his sister-in-law. Henriette Anne had been born at Exeter on 16 June 1644, the last child of Charles I and his French wife Henrietta Maria, whose sister-in-law the queen mother of France sent over the best mid-wife from France, Madame Peronne, for the delivery. France had a school for midwives, England did not, which made them very much in demand. In 1646 Henriette Anne

had to be smuggled out of the country dressed as a boy when the royalist cause had been lost, and she was brought up in France courtesy of the Regent, her aunt Anna Maria Mauritia of Austria, the queen mother. She was only 17 when she was married to Monsieur, and since he made no secret of the fact that he did not love women, although he managed to get her pregnant regularly, it is not surprising that the lively young princess, the favourite sister of Charles II, who called her Minette, should enjoy being courted by Louis XIV. The matter became patent on 23 July 1661 when they both performed in the court *Ballet des Saisons*, with Henriette Anne dressed as Diana goddess of the chase, and Louis XIV dressed as Spring sinking to his knees to hail her as the Queen of Beauty. Both queen mothers said that matters were going too far, and if Louis XIV must flirt when his poor wife was pregnant with their first child, he should select a maid of honour. He did: the shy, devout, timid Louise de La Vallière. Another scandal – the king had a mistress. Henriette Anne was piqued. The Spanish Queen Marie Thérèse, heavily pregnant with the Dauphin, had to puzzle out what was going on through the fog of French, but once the king started coming to bed in the middle of the night with the excuse that he had been working late, comprehension dawned. The Infanta may have been brought up like a nun but even she could see through that excuse, and she was deeply hurt. Fashion had to pause, for the queen, Henriette Anne and soon the royal mistress were all pregnant in loose gowns, and hairstyles became dominant.

Married women were expected to cover the hair with caps, and most of them did, but the court was different. Although the Church insisted on coverage it was in Italy that married women in high society had begun wearing lighter alternatives – veils, turbans, hairnets – from the early fourteenth century; in Spain decorated plaits were worn. The rise of Protestantism in the north, with its stress on modesty, gave a new

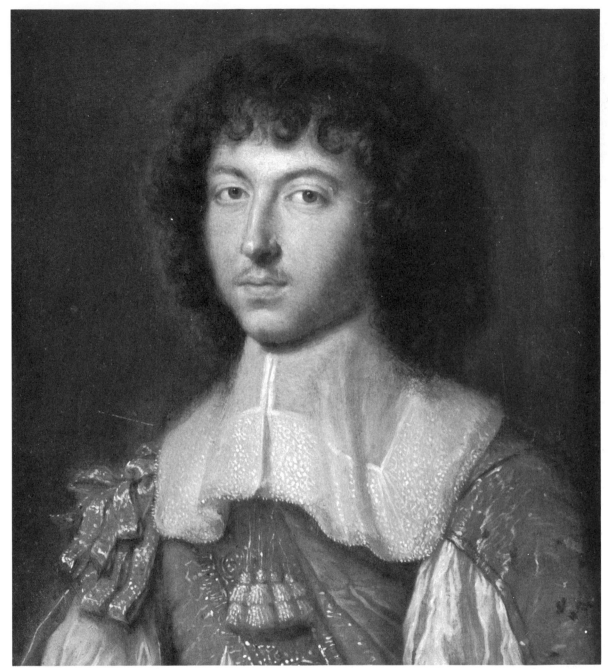

11 Wallerand Vaillant, 'Louis XIV', 1660.
The young king wears a cloth of silver doublet, ribbons and
a silver embroidered baldric. His hair was dark blond, his
eyes blue black, and his skin olive; he had an aquiline nose
and is here shown sporting his new moustache. He was now
flirting with his sister-in-law Henriette Anne of England.
(*Stockholm University Art Collection*)

12 Antoine Matthieu, 'Henriette Anne of England
Duchesse d'Orléans', 1664.
The first Madame sits with the portrait of her husband
Philippe, the king's brother, and is shown as mistress of the
arts which she loved in her short life. The loose dress and
sandals are the Roman timeless imperial image, but her
sleeves and hair are in the fashion of 1664. Henriette Anne
took part in many masquerades and plays but her health was
poor. (*Versailles, cliché des Musées Nationaux*)

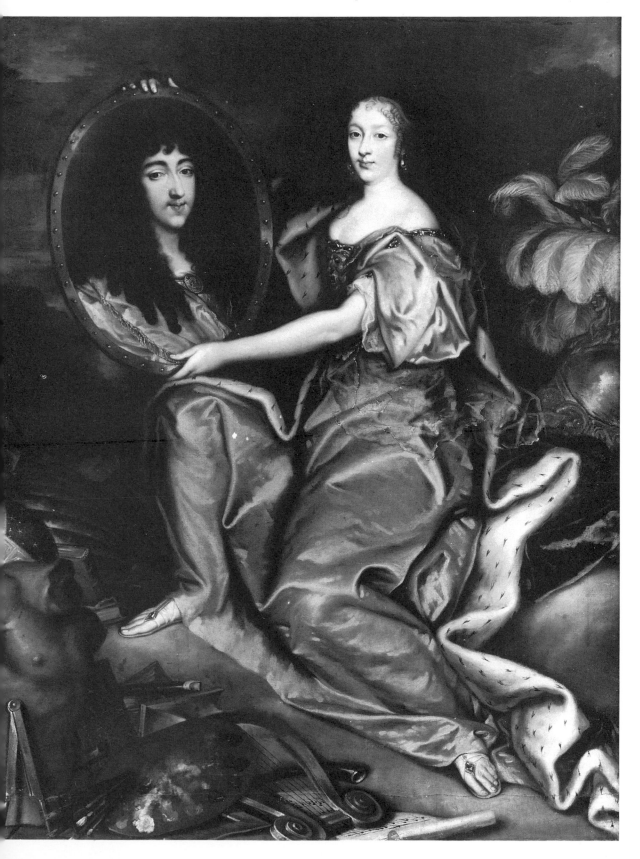

13 Pierre Mignard, 'Louise de La Vallière'.

The first official mistress of Louis XIV was chosen to keep him away from his sister-in-law. Shy and modest, Louise did not try to embarrass the queen Marie Thérèse who in time came to be friendly with her. Louise took the veil after a second mistress was appointed at court. She bore Louis XIV a son and a daughter. The wooden panel of the portrait has cracked. (*Musée des Beaux Arts, Marseilles*)

14 Sebastian Bourdon, 'Nicolas Fouquet Marquis de Belle-Ile, Comte de Melun et de Vaux'.

The superintendent of finances since 1653 had been chosen by Cardinal Mazarin. Ministers of the Crown were expected to wear black at the start of the reign, so the marquis is dressed in a black suit with just a hint of luxury in the black lace down the front of the doublet and the silver ribbon on the open sleeve, from which the shirt sleeve bursts. He wears his own hair and a waxed moustache like Louis XIV. The marquis's new palace, however, was richer and was to be his undoing. (*Versailles, cliché des Musées Nationaux*) importance to caps in the sixteenth century but the south still differed, with Emperor Charles V's wife Eleanor of Portugal wearing her hair in braids. In England caps received a blow when the virgin Queen Elizabeth I came to the throne, as she was not married and so did not have to wear a cap at all. English wives at court began to copy the queen's hairstyles, and dispensed with caps. The French court saw the de' Medici queens from Italy bringing the southern capless look with them, and so caps for married women disappeared from the English and French courts about the same time. This gave a new career to hairdressers. Frizzed and curled styles were the rage when Louis XIV was a boy, but by the late 1640s ringlets were coming into vogue. New styles were launched by the current queen and her ladies as part of the propaganda for the court as a leader of taste and to show its superiority over other courts. Accordingly, the ringlets were given even greater elaboration, with a cluster of at least half a dozen on each side of the face. Ear wires were invented to hold the ringlets out from the head. None have survived, but they were probably U-shaped over the head, and then stuck out at the sides so that the ringlets could be draped over them. Their stability was not very great and memoirs contain comments about ladies having to have their hairstyles adjusted and withdrawing in haste as a wire slipped. Hairpins were employed to anchor it, and the bun at the back gave a foundation, but the least knock on the projecting ringlets could dislodge the composition. By the middle of the 1660s the ringlets had become too common, so the court changed to puffs, where the side of the hair was puffed out, and the ringlets shortened. Gradually the puff grew bigger and the ringlets fewer so that by 1670 the puff was the dominant feature, and provided the new look for the next decade. For men the periwig was becoming increasingly important. Examples had been sported since 1656, but Louis XIV was very vain about his dark blond hair and did not adopt a full perruque until 1672. In England the English court adopted periwigs in 1663–4. The early versions were a mass of curls with a flat top, but by the later 1660s ringlets were cascading down many a man's face.

The next scandal was the arrest in September 1661 of the Superintendent of Finances, Nicolas Fouquet, Marquis de Belle-Ile, Comte de Melun et de Vaux. It was well known that Fouquet was building himself a splendid mansion at Vaux-le-Vicomte. In fact, Louis XIV approved of Fouquet engaging a French artist Le Brun for the décor, a French architect Le Vau for the building, and a French gardener Le Nôtre for the grounds, instead of Italians. The opening party was on 17 August for 6,000 guests and the king was astounded. He could not entertain 6,000 guests in such magnificence as this. Fouquet must have creamed off more than was usual from the royal finances. Louis XIV muttered to his mother: 'We must make these people disgorge!' Fouquet had done the unpardonable, he had made Louis XIV feel outclassed. He was arrested, and the tapestries, brocade curtains, silver ornaments, carved furniture, the statues in the gardens, and 1,000 orange trees, were transported to the royal châteaux. The trial lasted a long time for Fouquet was too clever for the judges, but the king wanted his condemnation, and Fouquet was sent off to the fortress at Pignerol until his death. A co-resident in that jail was the mysterious man in a velvet mask. The minister responsible for compiling the Crown's case was Jean Baptiste Colbert, Mazarin's general factotum, noted for his meanness, who was after Fouquet's job and now got it. People called him the North Wind. Yet even Colbert could not restrain the king when he now decided to expand Versailles to outshine Vaux-le-Vicomte. Colbert was appalled: surely the Louvre was big enough for any king; but the king would not listen. Le Vau, Le Nôtre and Le Brun were all directed to start improving Versailles.

The site was impossible:

The most sad and ungracious of all places, without a view, without woods, without water, without earth for it is either moving sand or marsh, without good air in consequence, which cannot be well. It pleased him to tyrannise nature, and to dominate her by force of art and money. He built everything one after the other, without a general design: the beautiful and the ugly were knitted together, the vast and the constricted too.[2]

This was the Duc de Saint Simon's opinion in the 1690s when the palace was gigantic. Colbert might wring his hands but Louis XIV was not interested in bills. He did not know what it would cost, because his idea of the grandeur he wanted kept increasing. The cost in human suffering was even greater. The speed and the marshy site caused many fatalities among the army of labourers, and the work continued for the remainder of the reign. Madame de Sevigné wrote on 12 October 1678:

The court is at St Cloud; the King wanted to go to Versailles on Saturday, but God, it seems, wished it not, by the impossibility of getting the buildings ready to receive him,

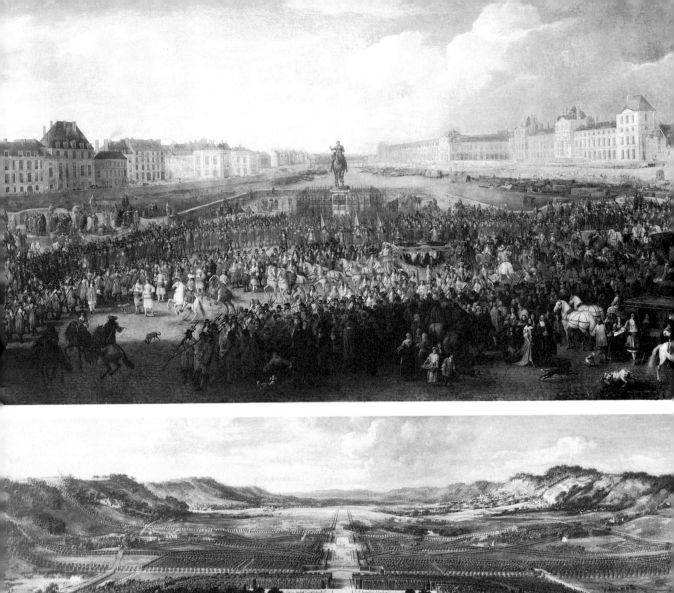

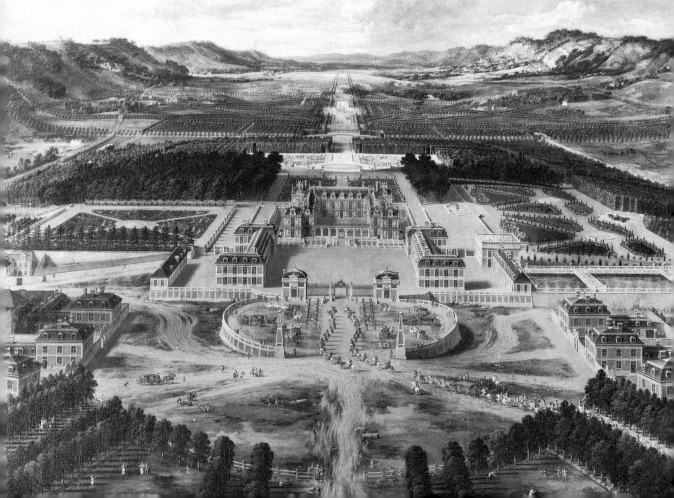

OPPOSITE ABOVE
15 Adam Franz van der Meulen, 'Louis XIV Crossing the Pont Neuf, Paris'.
Surrounded by guards the royal coach passes in front of the statue of Henri IV, Louis XIV's grandfather. On the right spreads the enormous Palace of the Louvre, which ministers thought big enough for any monarch; but Louis disliked cities. The man in the right-hand corner by the coach shows how the doublet was almost disappearing in front; the petticoat breeches form a full skirt, but much shorter than those worn by women. The hems of fine ladies can be seen sweeping the ground, but a working woman has them above the ankle. (*Musée des Beaux Arts, Grenoble*)

OPPOSITE BELOW
16 Pierre Patel, 'View of the Château of Versailles about 1668'.
Louis XIII's hunting lodge forms the core of the new palace, to which his son added pavilions and enlarged the formal gardens where the first fêtes at Versailles took place. Eventually most of the foreground was to disappear under Louis XIV's ever-expanding concept of a combination of a royal residence with hunting amenities. (*Versailles, cliché des Musées Nationaux*)

17 Adam Franz van der Meulen, 'Versailles under Construction', *c*. 1680.
The new controller general of finances, Colbert, in ministerial black with a hat, despaired of the ever-expanding palace. Up to 36,000 labourers were engaged on the building and landscaping while the Army was called in to excavate the canals. The church at the left was to be swept away, and so were Louis XIV's first constructions. (*Reproduced by Gracious Permission of Her Majesty the Queen*)

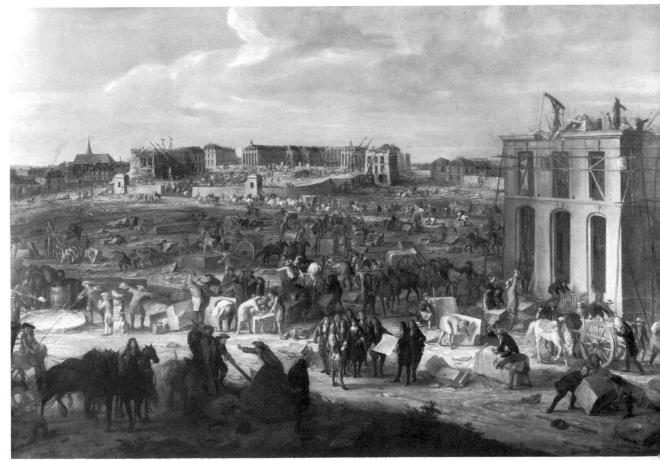

and by the prodigious mortality of the workmen – every night wagon fulls of the dead are carried out, as from the Hôtel Dieu. This melancholy step is concealed as much as possible, in order not to alarm the other workmen, and to decry the air of this unworthy favourite.[3]

Protests were not allowed. An old woman whose labourer son was killed on the site called the king a tyrant in her grief, and was flogged in public. A few days later an old man of 60 who also complained about the death of a son was sent to the galleys, where he would not last long, and had his tongue cut out. Councillor d'Ormesson commented that this was a new use of that punishment. Tongues were normally cut out only for blasphemy, but now it seemed that to criticize Louis XIV was a sin too.

The man responsible for the royal image was Charles Le Brun, and since Louis XIV considered himself the equal of emperors, the imperial impression was enforced by portraying the king as an ancient Roman emperor, even when recording his contemporary exploits. Le Brun was to decorate the great gallery at Versailles with murals of the king as a Roman conqueror. This was very much in accordance with the latest artistic policy that had come from Italy. So far as establishing an eternal image was concerned, ancient Roman armour, free of the date-stamp of contemporary fashion, was the ideal, while the ladies could be portrayed in nightgowns of a classical looseness. Charles Perrault singled out for special praise one series painted by Le Brun for the king:

no body hath ever represented all sorts of Subjects with more of *Nature* and *Becomingness*, nor better observ'd what the Masters of the Art call *Le Costume*. To be convinc'd of this, a Man need only see the five great *Tableaux* he has done of *The History of Alexander*, and particularly that of the Family of *Darius*: where the Airs of the Head speak no less the several Countrys of the Persons there represented, than their *Habillements* faithfully design'd upon the Antique.[4]

The official image on coins, statutary, proclamations, seals, and in art, became Roman.

Strangely enough, when Councillor d'Ormesson had dinner with Le Brun on 15 November 1665 he found him sadly disenchanted. Le Brun still felt very loyal to his first major patron Fouquet and detested the harshness with which he had been treated. The age was too hard. The demands upon himself were enormous and he never received any thanks, while people were jealous of his position with the king. Le Brun had begun as an artist of great promise. His *Hercules and Diomedes*, for example (Nottingham

Castle Museum), is full of Baroque vitality and movement, but once all the responsibilities of the royal image and all the decorations, furniture, tapestries, silverware and décor at Versailles descended upon his shoulders, the life went out of his work.

The first great festivity at Versailles was held in the park on 11 June 1664. It was called the 'Divertissemens des Deux Reines', as both Queen Marie Thérèse, and the queen mother attended, with the current queen of the king's heart, Louise de La Vallière.

An amphitheatre for 200 spectators was set up among the trees and lit by chandeliers. After a flourish of trumpets and a clash of cymbals the Sun God Apollo, attired in gold and azure blue, entered in his chariot, escorted by paladins. He was joined by the Times, the Seasons and the Hours. The court composer J.B. Lully led in the musicians for the procession of the Seasons with Spring on a Spanish horse, Summer on an elephant, Autumn on a camel, and Winter on a bear, each with its followers – 12 gardeners, 12 sowers, 12 vintage workers, and 12 old men. After a ballet of heroes in Roman armour, the four controllers of the royal household entered as Abundance, Joy, Good Cheer and Cleanliness to oversee the arrival of a table loaded with delicacies for the ladies. On the second day there was a Molière comedy with dancing and music, and on the third a ballet at ten in the evening. The poet Marigny wrote the description, to notify the civilized world of the glamorous glory of the court of France, if one did not look below the surface.[5]

One foreigner who came to see the splendours was the Italian abbot Sebastiano Locatelli. On 11 November 1664 he saw Louis XIV going to mass at St Germain l'Auxerois, dressed in a black velvet suit of doublet and petticoat breeches with a large floral pattern, and with the silver star of the Saint Esprit on his cloak, in the same way as the knights of Malta wore their crosses. He carried a short cane and wore a small hat with a rose of diamonds at one side. It was unusual for a man of his rank not to be wearing a periwig, but his long, dark blond hair was still plentiful. His height was heroic. The dukes and peers were dressed more richly than the king, but his mother had always stressed a modest appearance in church. When in Paris Queen Marie Thérèse always went to mass at Notre Dame de Lorette. She wore a brocade gown flaming with great silver flowers, but modestly asked her page to drop her train inside the church. Locatelli thought her beautiful with her very pale skin, blue

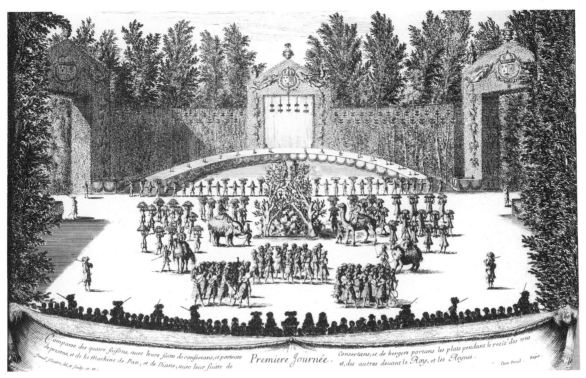

Comparse des quatre saisons, avec leurs suitte de confestans, et porteurs de present, et de la Machine de Pan, et de Diane, avec leur suitte de **Première Journée** *Consertans, et de bergers portans les plats pendant le recit des Vers et, des autres devant le Roy, et les Reynes.*

18 F. Chauveau, 'The First Day of the Pleasures of the Enchanted Island', 1673.
The parade of the Four Seasons during the celebrations mounted in honour of the two official queens and the royal mistress in 1664, which was not published with illustrations until 1673. Each Season was mounted on a different beast, and examples of produce were carried on the heads of the followers. The whole series of extravaganzas at Versailles was designed to impress the world, hence the publications about them. (*The British Library*)

eyes and curly blond hair, and could not understand why Louis XIV had to be so blind as to take a mistress of only ordinary good looks. Locatelli saw La Vallière in the park having her hairstyle adjusted which suggests the wires had slipped. He was able to attend the queen's dressing at the Louvre. While the ladies did her hair in ringlets, she sat in a well-boned white corset and a narrow silk skirt. He was amazed that male tailors brought her dress, a rich fabric with alternating flowers in blue and gold upon a silver ground, and even put it on her and laced it up. The ladies placed the jewellery on her hair and corsage. The queen was shorter than in church, as she was only wearing slippers, not high-heeled shoes. She said not a word but pointed when she wanted anything, as her French was still limited. Once dressed she hurried off to the queen mother to chat in Spanish.

Locatelli looked at Versailles where three avenues to Paris 21 miles long had just been begun, which would involve levelling some hills. The amount of labour involved was beyond imagining, thousands of men with picks and shovels, wheelbarrows and carts, like ants. He got the opportunity to see Louis XIV in his glory when the king reviewed his army on the plain of St Denis on 6 April 1665. The Swiss Guard were there, all tall, in their uniforms of red and blue frieze, decorated with braid, and tufts of silk and silver, with black bonnets trimmed with red, white and blue plumes. Three hundred Grand Musketeers, on white or dappled horses, wore blue riding cassocks embroidered back and front with the royal cypher in gold of crosses with sun rays, over very fine camlet coats decked with silver embroidery. The horse caparisons were embroidered with suns in silver at the corners, because Louis XIV had taken the motto 'Ubique Solus' with the sun as his device. Three hundred Lesser Musketeers wore drugget tabards and coats with no silver, but their horses' caparisons bore the initial L surmounted by a crown in gold. These all constituted the royal guard. The infantry consisted of 120 companies all in grey uniforms, the cloth for which was one of England's biggest standing export orders. Colbert would change that. There were also 15 companies in red and 15 in blue, as well as

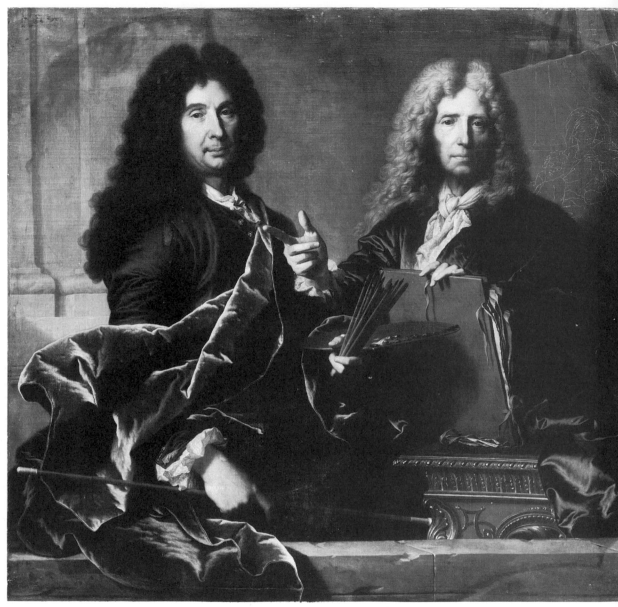

19 Hyacinthe Rigaud, 'Charles Le Brun and Pierre Mignard'.

Two court artists portrayed by a third. Le Brun was director of the new Royal Academy of Painting and Sculpture and of the Gobelins tapestry manufactory, and designer for all the interiors and sculptures at Versailles. Mignard was his rival and a fashionable portraitist. The royal visual image was Le Brun's responsibility; he represented Louis XIV in Roman armour as a hero outclassing Alexander the Great. Literary propaganda was the responsibility of the Petite Académie with Racine and Quinault among its members. Louis XIV was the first king to have a permanent propaganda machine. (*The Louvre, cliché des Musées Nationaux*)

2,000 cavalry. The king was attended by 22 dukes, and was most noticeable with his flame-coloured hat, and his hair held back by two big ribbons in flame. He wore a cravat of Venetian lace over a gold collar, and a coat of clear blue moiré (mohair) so covered with gold and silver embroidery it was hardly visible beneath. The coat was worn unbuttoned to display a vest of brocade and gold in the Polish style, fastened with large golden galloons, and decked with large diamonds. A sash went around his waist in the antique manner and was fastened by two gold lilies with two diamonds gleaming at the tops. The kneebreeches were in walloon drugget with flame-coloured garters covered in gold embroidery. His stockings were tobacco-toned, as were his shoes of English calfskin. The spurs were in violet steel, enamelled, and fastened on with gold buckles encrusted with diamonds. King Sun literally sparkled and gleamed.[6]

The coat and vest were the newest combination. Overcoats had been worn all the century, but about 1660 someone had the idea of wearing a coat instead of a doublet over his shirt. As doublets had got so short he probably felt the need for something offering more cover. Moreover, in the army the buff coats that were lighter than full armour had been growing longer during the 1650s, to offer better protection for the legs, and this too suggested a longer look than doublets. In London Samuel Pepys noted that gentlemen started to wear coats in 1661, and now Louis XIV had taken them up. He did not discard doublets and petticoat breeches completely but wore them for more official occasions as an older kind of

suit, and bridegrooms continued to wear them for weddings up to the 1690s.

The novelty was the Polish-style vest under the coat. Locatelli used the term *zimarra* which means an ankle-length garment as worn by Turks under the caftan. The vest worn by Louis was not so long as his kneebreeches and garters were clearly visible, so Locatelli may have been thinking of the cut and the sash more than the length. Certainly Turkish styles

---

20 S. de Saint-André, 'The Two Queens of France'.
The queen mother on the left wears Roman-type armour to commemorate her defeat of the Fronde when she was Regent. Her niece and daughter-in-law Queen Marie Thérèse has fruit and leaves to indicate her pregnancy. She bore Louis XIV six children but only the eldest son survived. The death of the queen mother from cancer of the breast in 1666 robbed the childlike queen of her best friend and compatriot. They spoke to each other in Spanish, which Louis XIV could also speak having learned it from his mother. (*Versailles, cliché des Musées Nationaux*)

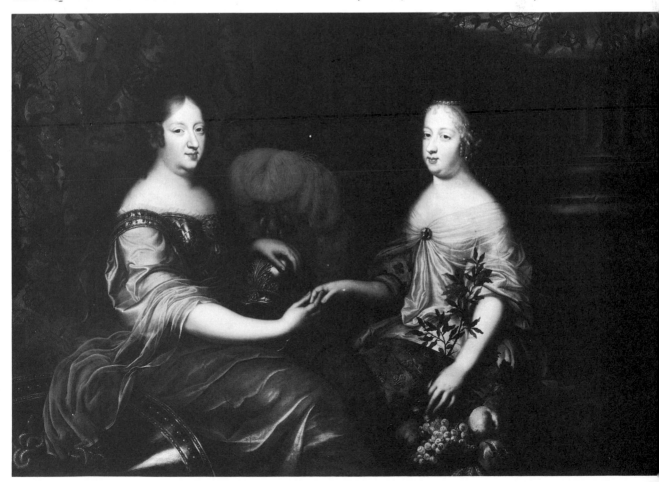

could find their way to Paris worn by Poles, given the close relationship between the Polish queen and the French court. The short Polish jackets may have been the inspiration behind the wearing of vests under coats, and many French and Dutch men started wearing them, until the English changed the suit. Vests reached to the top of the hips, whence the petticoat breeches flared out, and the result was too fussy for English tastes.

The court had to go into mourning in 1665. Louis XIV broke his promise to his father-in-law not to attack Spain, by sending French troops to help Portugal to beat the Spanish. The shock killed Philip IV, and two queens of France mourned the loss of a brother and a father. The queen mother said to Madame de Motteville that her son was cold and indifferent to the feelings of others. On 20 January 1666 the queen mother herself died of cancer of the breast after years of pain, and little Marie Thérèse lost her best friend at court. Monsieur Philippe made the greatest display of grief, and Louis wept all night, but this did not prevent him from officially demanding the Spanish Netherlands from the new king of Spain, Carlos II, his wife's half brother, an action which his mother would have deplored.

The Marquis de Saint Maurice, envoy from Duke Charles Emmanuel II of Savoy, reached France in 1667 as the military preparations to seize the Spanish Netherlands were in full flood. He saw Louis XIV at Compiègne on 13 July and observed that he spent an hour and a half a day getting dressed, of which half an hour was devoted to waxing his moustache in front of the mirror, even when he was with the army. All the mourning had stopped display for the time being, but the marquis thought the royal levée at the Louvre was the most beautiful court picture in the world: three rooms full of people of quality, and 800 coaches in the courtyard. He saw the Dauphin now aged six, who had been breeched and wore a coat and periwig like an adult, although he was told what to say by his governess Madame la Maréchale de la Mothe-Houdancourt. When he was seven the Duc de Montaussier would take over as governor. The invasion began in 1668, and the whole court set off after the army – the queen, the mistress now created a duchess since the queen mother's death, and a new challenger for the post of royal mistress, Athenaïs Pardaillon de Gondrin Marquise de Montespan, who was blond, with huge azure eyes, an aquiline nose, small mouth, good teeth, and was ambitious, calculating and arrogant in ways that Louise de La

Vallière was not. The king and his harem, joked the troops.

As it happened the Marquis de Montespan strongly objected to his wife's pursuit of the king. He had written to her on 15 May 1665: 'The more magnificent the Court is, the more uneasy do I become. Wealth and opulence are needed there, and to your family I never figured as a Croesus.'[7] His wife had had four years as a lady of the palace so now it was time to return to her husband in Provence. He wrote that the estates were overflowing with luscious peaches, strawberries and raspberries. The handsome king might be the favourite of all the ladies, but there would always be ten to replace her. This stung. The Marquise de Montespan did not intend to be replaced by anybody and succeeded in seducing the king. Her husband refused the title of duke to keep him quiet, and started proceedings for a legal separation, sent the bailiffs to reclaim his coach while his wife was in it, and put his servants into mourning. Further he ordered Athenaïs to stop using his livery and coat of arms. Louis XIV suggested she have a livery of orange and silver but she chose dark blue and gold. This was unprecedented, a wife's servants not wearing the husband's family colours, and made the relationship very obvious. Thus Louis XIV now had a wife and two mistresses, but Montespan with her love of jewellery and luxurious clothes was better at making the court sparkle than either the queen or La Vallière. The latter endured the situation until 1674 then she became a Carmelite nun, the queen herself handing her the veil at the service, for she had come to prefer the quiet Louise to the ruthless Montespan.

Town after town in the Spanish Netherlands succumbed before the French attack in 1668. Louis ordered victory celebrations at Versailles in July, and the court rushed to spend money. Some spent 15,000 livres on French lace. One merchant sold 80,000 livres of lace. The Marquis de Saint Maurice bemoaned that it cost him almost 4,000 livres to dress his wife, children and himself for the festivities, but he consoled himself with the thought that when one is among fools one must be foolish oneself[8]. The Marquis de Montespan had been right to worry about the expense of life at court. Louis wanted the aristocracy to spend its all, as Saint Simon was well aware:

He loved above all splendour, magnificence, profusion. This taste he turned into a political maxim, and inspired his whole court to adopt it. It was to please him that one had to throw oneself into gambling, into clothes, into carriages, into buildings and gaming. These were the occasions when he spoke to people. The result was that he tried and succeeded to squeeze the whole world into putting luxury as a point of honour, and for some parties a necessity, and so little by little reduced society to depend entirely upon his favours to survive. Furthermore a court superb in all it did, was satisfaction to his pride.[9]

The following Christmas Louis XIV told Saint Maurice that he had just decided to build a town at Versailles to service the palace. In this haphazard way Versailles grew. By now even the Sultan of Turkey had heard about Versailles and he sent an envoy on 5 December 1669. Louis XIV donned a coat covered with diamonds which had cost 14,000,000 livres, and Monsieur's coat was embroidered with pearls and jewels. Twenty Turkish horsemen had robes of green serge and dirty turbans, and the ambassador wore a garment of red camlet, with no silk or gold in sight. The only splendour lay in the golden bag containing the Sultan's letter. The envoy was furious when Louis

XIV refused to stand to receive the imperial communication and said it was an insult to the Sublime Porte, but Louis considered himself the equal of emperors, although he was to be a conqueror only of towns and counties, not continents.[10]

The English court could not fail to notice all these goings on. Its own queen mother was French, and Charles II had spent much of his exile there, when he had acquired a French tailor Claude Sourceau. He wrote to Henriette Anne in April 1660: 'I have sent to Sourceau to make me some clothes for the summer, and I have given him orders to bring you some ribbon so that you may choose the trimming and the feathers.'[11] Having a sister at the French court was very useful and on 14 September 1668 Charles II wrote to thank her for some scented gloves: 'They are as good as is possible to smell.' He tried to divide the office of royal tailor of the robes into two, with Sourceau in Paris starting clothes and the London tailors John Allen and William Watts finishing them; this was done with the coronation clothes in 1661. They cost £2,271 19s 10d but Charles II could not spend money as freely as his cousin Louis, for his kingdoms were much smaller and he had Parliament to contend with; in 1662 Sourceau and Allen and Watts were still petitioning for payment for that coronation outfit. Similarly, the first Earl of Sandwich had a London tailor Mr Pim, but for his coronation suit sent the order to a Paris tailor, which cost him

21 French School, 'The Embassy to King Charles II of England made by Monseigneur the Prince de Ligne', 1660. Charles II and the ambassador both had French tailors, and the suite displays French fashion at its extreme with tiny doublets, voluminous petticoat breeches, huge knee ruffles and ostrich-plumed hats. In 1666 the English court would revolt against the domination of French fashion. (*Copyright ACL Brussels; photograph by courtesy of the Prince de Ligne, Beloeil*)

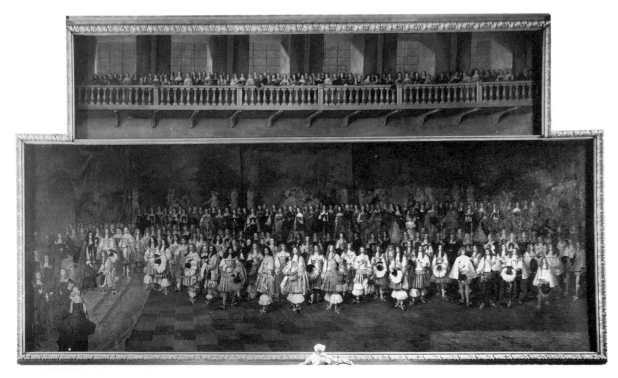

£200. The same pattern existed in the Spanish Netherlands, for in 1660 Philip IV asked the Prince de Ligne to visit London on his behalf to congratulate Charles II on his restoration. The Prince then sent a gentleman of his household, Sieur de Blondel, to Paris to oversee the making of two rich suits for the prince and his son the Marquis de Roubaix. The rest of his suite were dressed by Brussels tailors. The embassy landed at Gravesend and for the entry into London put its 70 members into pink liveries decorated with silver galloons and yellow ones. The doublets were yellow satin with a floral pattern, and the cloaks were lined with the same satin and decorated up to the collar. All had silk sleeves and plumed hats. The trumpeters' cassocks were in flame-coloured velvet with the same decorations and bouquets of plumes, and their bandeliers were embroidered. Twenty-four lackeys were dressed the same, and the 20 palfreys had caparisons embroidered with the arms and motto of the Prince de Ligne.

The second livery was worn for the public audience at Whitehall Palace when the prince had 12 pages in cloaks and petticoat breeches in flame-coloured velvet edged with yellow velvet, and a galloon of silver on each side. The doublets were cloth of silver as was the lining of the cloaks, and the doublets were overlaid with gold and silver lace. All wore silk stockings and plumed hats. The trumpeters were also in flame velvet. The 20 lackeys, two valets, and two Swiss Guards were dressed in pink cloth, edged with strips of yellow velvet and silver galloons. M. Neuville, the third of the 12 gentlemen in the domestic suite, wrote that it was impossible to imagine anything more rich and better ordered.[12]

A walking advertisement for French fashion at the English court was the Comte de Gramont whose valet Termes was a trans-Channel commuter, being sent by the count to bring suits, and gifts for the ladies from Paris. Perfumed gloves, pocket looking-glasses, apricot paste, scents, ornate boxes, were typical. Even Pepys knew a French agent, W. Batelier, who brought books, clothes, gloves, shoes and hoods from Paris. Aristocratic gentlemen on the Grand Tour would receive orders from uncles, aunts, brothers and sisters to pick up hats, fans, gloves, lace and silks, in Paris. It was not necessary to go that far however, for Marie and Thomas Cheret ran a successful French shop at Covent Garden. Pepys called there in 1664 for a mask, and the Cherets are also named in the clothing accounts of the Earls of Northumberland, and the

Duchess of Lauderdale, and in 1690 were selling to Mary II. They offered lace bands, lace cuffs, hatbands, orange and jasmine scented gloves, French hoods, French colbertine lace, gauze scarves. The gloves varied in price from plain ones at 2s 6d, to scented frangipani and jasmine, 5s 6d, to the most expensive gloves by Martial of Paris at 30s. There were French people inside Whitehall Palace, for Pepys bought some hair pieces for his wife from the Queen's tire-woman Madame Gotiers in 1669, and in 1671 Evelyn encountered a 'French peddling woman, one *Madame de boord*, that used to bring petticoats, & fanns & baubles out of France to the Ladys'. Pepys's perruquier was Monsieur Robbins who also ran a French eating house. The royal staff included two French composers and ten French dancing masters.[13] There was so much French influence in fact that it led to protest. John Evelyn wrote his *Tyrannus; or, The Mode* in 1661 and gave a copy to Charles II. Why, he asked, did the English have to dance to a French tailor's tune? Why copy all the fashions of that mercurial nation? 'would the great Persons of *England* but owne their Nation, and assert themselves as they ought to do, by making choice of some Virile, and comely Fashion, which should incline to neither extream, and be constant to it, 'twould prove of infinite more reputation to us, then now there is . . .'[14] French styles were too effete with all the ribbons, petticoat breeches, high-heeled shoes and scented gloves. The poet Samuel Butler penned his *Satire upon our Ridiculous Imitation of the French* about 1663, saying that his countrymen were monkeys to copy every affectation from Paris. At Oxford Anthony à Wood complained that the decay of learning was due to the English copying French follies. The importation began to worry Parliament and in 1662 it banned the import of foreign bone lace, cut work, embroidery, fringe, band-strings, buttons and needle work. The City protested that French fashion was bad for English industries and told Charles II to act. In October 1665 Lord Arlington wrote to the Lord Mayor that once the mourning for Philip IV of Spain was over, the king would only wear English manufactures in future, except for linen and calico, the Queen and court would do the same, and he wished the country to copy. This was only after the great plague of that year, and the clergy were telling the king that it was divine judgement upon his sinful court, for copying Catholic France, and a result of his immoral conduct. In 1666 the Great Fire of London was interpreted as further divine punishment so

Charles II decided he had better take the matter seriously and heed Evelyn's booklet on founding a national style. The name of Claude Sourceau had disappeared from the state papers after 1662, so he may have found the non-payment of bills and the distance too much to cope with. It was John Allen and William Watts, the king's English tailors, who now had to join with Charles II to devise something English. They agreed that the way Louis XIV wore his coat over his vest and petticoat breeches was too fussy, for it caused the petticoats to bunch in front. Charles II expressed a preference for narrow breeches as worn in Spain, without petticoats, which should produce a cleaner line. It was still felt, however, that a way to conceal the breeches would be more moral, so the idea of lengthening the vest was born. The English three-piece suit was created with the vest and the coat of equal lengths to the knee, worn over narrow Spanish breeches. This was a much simpler line that

the beribboned excesses of French style, and the English court launched it in October 1666. The first vests were plain, but by the queen's birthday ball on 15 November, cloth-of-silver vests appeared at £100

---

22 *Almanach Royal*, 1667, 'Louis XIV with the Ladies of the Court'.

In 1666 the English court introduced a reformed suit with the long coat and a long vest (waistcoat), discarding petticoat breeches and shrunken doublets completely. The engraving shows that Louis XIV tried the new look in 1667, for it had to be approved for publication. His coat and vest are not knee length but he has gone some way towards the English style, and so has his son the Dauphin aged six, who has been breeched into an English-type suit. The queen under the canopy is probably accompanied by Henriette Anne, Duchesse d'Orléans, and the king's cousin Anne Marie Louise, Duchesse de Montpensier. Their hairstyles show the puff beginning to oust ringlets. Bare necklines were the height of fashion and *de rigueur* at court. (*Versailles, cliché des Musées Nationaux*)

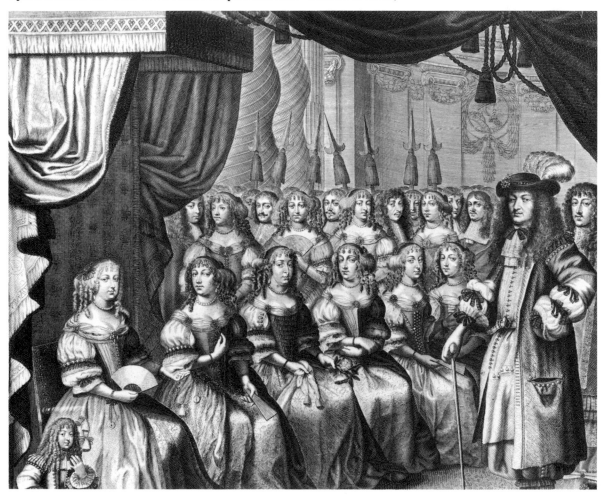

each, while others were even richer, being embroidered with jewels in the French manner. The country followed eagerly, for long vests were anti-French and anti-Catholic.

Louis XIV was not amused. How dare little Britannia try to diminish his glory by inventing fashions of her own! Reports that he put his servants into English vests were not substantiated, and sufficient illustrations survive from 1667 to show that Louis XIV actually tried longer vests on himself, not completely to the knee like the English, but to above the knee, and he cut down on the ribbons. Yet the simplicity was too modest. He had his coats and vests covered with gold and silver embroidery but he seems to have missed the swing of petticoat breeches, the burst of white linen beneath the little doublets, and reverted to them by 1671. Of course in summer they were ideal, but in cooler weather coats and vests were

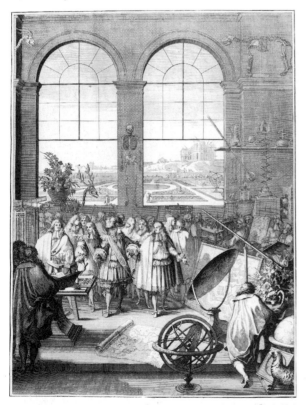

23 S. Le Clerc, engraved Goyton, 'Louis XIV visiting the Academy of Sciences', 1671; from Claude Perrault's *Mémoires pour servir à l'histoire naturelle des animaux*. Louis XIV reverted to petticoat breeches and wore them with a very short coat, which the English laughed at. He was too fond of the ribbons, the swirling skirts, the lavish linen, for the restraint of the English style to affect him yet, although it would do so in time. (*The British Library*)

an improvement, so they continued to spread despite Louis XIV's doubts. He decided on a counter-attack. He was already planning to send his sister-in-law Henriette Anne Duchesse d'Orléans to England to persuade her brother Charles II to desert the Protestant Triple Alliance between England, the Netherlands and Sweden, for Louis XIV wanted to attack the Dutch without her allies interfering. He now instructed the duchesse to laugh the English out of their vests as well, and saw her off with a suite of over 200 persons. The English did not care for the French style – 'The French Court wearing then Excessive *short lac'd Coats*: some Scarlet some Blew with Broad wast *Belts*' – and the comic actor Nokes guyed the French short coat in Shadwell's *The Impertinents*, when the Duke of Monmouth lent him his sword and belt 'on purpose to ape the French'.[15] The performance was at Canterbury. Negotiations were carried on at Dover Castle, while Louis XIV waited for developments at Dunkirk. He offered Charles II £160,000 to declare himself a Catholic, and a subsidy of 3,000,000 livres a year (£200,000) to go to war against the Netherlands. Henriette Anne charmed her brother into acceptance, and returned to France in June 1670 as a heroine, to Monsieur Philippe's intense jealousy. By the end of that month Henriette Anne was dead. Poisoned by Monsieur's homosexual friends, was the first thought of many, and the Duke of Buckingham wanted to declare war on France. Nowadays acute peritonitis is proposed. She was 26. Did she persuade Charles II to give up long vests? Briefly perhaps. He was painted in 1671 in a coat and short vest of the French type, but by a Flemish artist. Vests did not vanish. The hip-length one was well established on the Continent and there are many examples in Dutch portraits. The British continued wearing long ones, and by 1678 the French had given up trying to resist for they began showing long English vests in the engravings of male fashion by St Jean. Louis XIV lost this round.

The long vest was not the only English fashion to influence the French. When Charles II launched his vest in 1666 his queen Catherine of Braganza announced that she would launch a fashion for women by shortening skirts. She raised the hem just enough to show the shoe, which kept skirts out of the dirt. This fashion spread rapidly, and the French ambassador Courtin sent the French court a full description:

There is nothing neater than the feet and ankles of the English ladies in their well-fitting shoes and silk stockings.

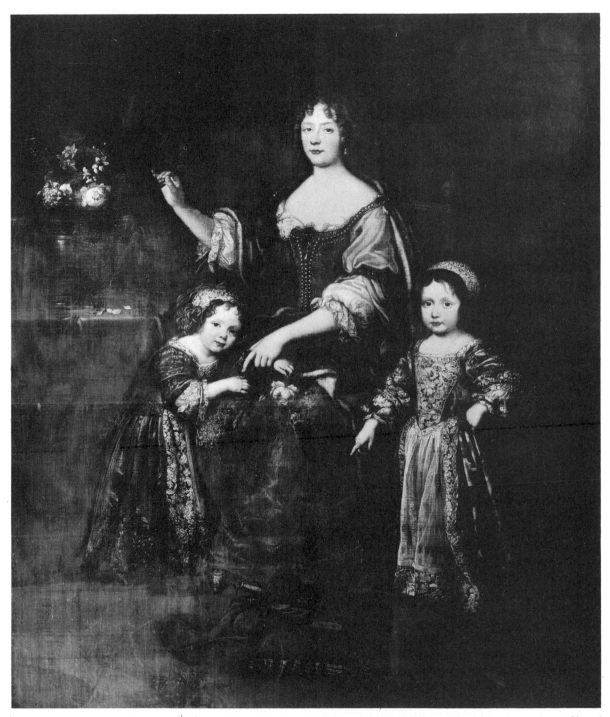

24 Attributed to Pierre Mignard, 'Elisabeth Charlotte of the Rhineland Palatinate Duchesse d'Orléans with her children'.

The new Madame, who married the king's brother Philippe in 1671 and became an invaluable reporter of events at Versailles, which she found an absurd institution. Her son Philippe Duc de Chartres, on the right, was to be the future Regent when Louis XIV died, and her daughter Elisabeth Charlotte was to marry the Duke of Lorraine in 1698. Their son Franz of Lorraine would marry the Empress Maria Theresia of Austria in 1736. (*Reproduced by Gracious Permission of Her Majesty the Queen*)

They wear their skirts short: and I often see legs so well turned that a sculptor would like to mould them. Green silk stockings are modish. The garter, of which glimpses are often afforded, is below the knee, and in black velvet with diamond buckles. Those who have no silk stockings to wear show a white skin smooth as satin. English women prefer being stockingless to wearing clumsy and disfiguring hosiery.[16]

In other words they were sexually attractive, so bold ladies like Louis XIV's new mistress the Marquise de Montespan were quick to copy. Short skirts became the dominant fashion for women until 1678 when long hems made a comeback, but of course there was an overlap into the 1680s.

Much to Louis XIV's relief the French hairdresser Martin was able to save the reputation of the French court by devising a new hairstyle for ladies in 1671, *l'hurlu brelu*. On 4 April 1671 the Marquise de Sevigné wrote to her daughter the Comtesse de Grignan that Madame Martin was promoting the new coiffure with excess:

Imagine a head parted in the middle like a peasant to within two fingers of the pad. The hair is cut on each side, stage by stage, to form large round curls with a negligent air, which do not come any lower than one finger below the ear. It looks very young and very pretty, like two bouquets of hair on each side. It is important not to cut the hair too short.

Ribbons are added in the ordinary way, and a large curl placed between the pad and the coiffure. Sometimes it hangs down to the throat. I do not know if I have represented this fashion very well for you: I'll have a doll's hair dressed to send to you.[17]

In January 1672 an attempt to launch a magazine about fashion and the court was made in Paris with *Le Mercure Galant*. John Dancer produced an English version, but it lacked sufficient funding to continue. It noted the vogue for green silk stockings, and said the big news was long-waisted gowns, with the waistline dropped to the hips. Men's coats were cut to show the low waist as well and the look was emphasized by wearing a broad sash at hip level. The king's taste for lavish embroidery showed in the wearing of coats laced or embroidered with gold and silver, while gold hatbands were ousting silk ones.

Charles II had taken a great fancy to a baby-faced girl in his sister's entourage, Louise de Keroualle. Louis XIV sent her back in 1671 fully equipped to be a royal mistress and French spy, with her hair cut in the hurlu brelu, and low-waisted French gowns. She was bedded at Euston Palace, and her stocking flung as if she had been a bride, reported Evelyn in disgust.

Notwithstanding the insult, the queen Catherine of Braganza adopted the shorter hairstyle. Louise was created Duchess of Portsmouth and soon proved very extravagant.

A very different lady arrived at the French court in 1671. Monsieur Philippe was given a new wife, Elisabeth Charlotte, daughter of the Elector of the Rhineland Palatinate. The wedding took place at Châlons on 21 November 1671. Saint Simon wrote that she was built like a Swiss Guard, and she adored hunting. Beside her Monsieur looked like a doll, but he managed to sire three children by her, of whom two survived. Madame Elisabeth Charlotte was not interested in fashion, but she wrote invaluable accounts about it back to her family. She preferred to wear her hunting habit all day in the scarlet livery of the royal hunt. Her German fondness for furs was laughed at by the French court. She upset the Marquise de Montespan by mocking her way of decorating her hurlu brelu hairstyle with diamonds and bejewelled pins. The new duchess was only 19 and had had a spartan upbringing, as her father Charles Louis was extremely mean. His sister-in-law had to intervene to ensure that Elisabeth Charlotte arrived in France with more than six shifts to her name. A dozen at least, she insisted. Accordingly the new Madame d'Orléans was very critical of French excess, the wearing of so much gold and silver at court, and kept herself aloof, being very proud of her German and English royal blood, for she was the granddaughter of James I's daughter Elisabeth, queen of Bohemia. But in December 1676 she suddenly found herself in the fashion. When hunting with the king her horse bolted and threw her. Louis XIV rushed to help her up and escorted her back to Versailles. The court decided that she was now in favour, so all the ladies started to copy Madame's fur tippets. How mad, Elisabeth Charlotte wrote home. They laughed at my furs in 1671 but in 1676 the *palatine* is the rage, all because the king likes me! This accidental invention of a fashion was to be repeated, for much depended on the king approving of someone and their style or idea.[18]

In 1673 the Comte de Saint Mayol, Jean Baptiste Primi Visconti, went to inspect the famous court of Louis XIV. He arrived just as the king, sword in hand and wearing boots as if he were off to the hunt, rode to Parlement and informed it that in future it could no longer license his laws. His signature alone would suffice. He did not have the courtesy to address the Parlement in his coronation suit and robes. Visconti

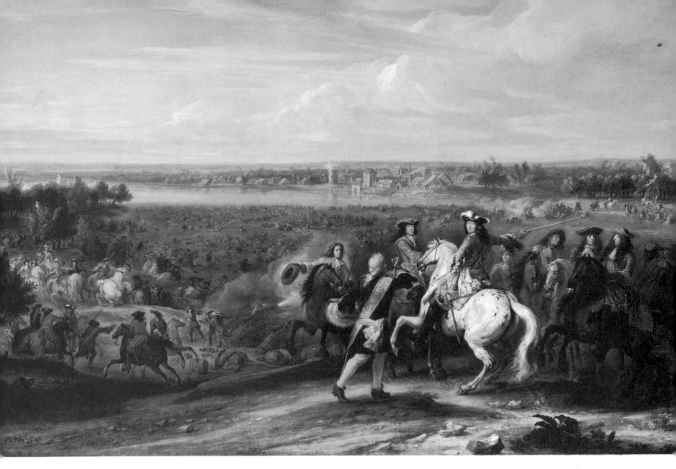

found that the king kept regular hours. His old nurse woke him at 8 a.m., he spend 10 to 12.30 p.m. with his councils for domestic, foreign and ecclesiastical affairs, then went to mass with the queen, and dined at 2 p.m. in public. The rest of the day was spent hunting or promenading through the grounds, and the evenings were occupied with cards, gaming, comedies and balls. Supper was at 11, after which he went to his mistress, but still ended up in the queen's bed for morning. The comte found Versailles too big, and it still was incomplete. He said the king was like an actor. He could be relaxed in private, but before appearing in front of the court he changed his expression and attitude to one of grandeur. Officials had been stripped of any decision making, and even generals and admirals had to refer to the king during action, which was time-consuming and impractical. Provincial governors had to reside at court. Nobody was trusted. The sight of the king leaving one of his castles with the bodyguard, the coaches, courtiers, horsemen, and the multitude of grooms and footmen running after him with much noise, was like a queen bee leaving the hive.

Visconti estimated that there were 7,000 servants and 4,000 Swiss and French guards plus halbediers

25 Adam Franz van der Meulen, 'Louis XIV Crossing the Rhine 12 June 1672'.
Not content with attacking the Hapsburgs, Louis now turned on the House of Orange by invading the Netherlands. However, he always led from the rear and avoided dangerous situations. His coat is smothered with embroidery, probably in gold, for even at the scene of battle King Sun could not look plain. The variety in cocking the hat shows the freedom which existed before the eighteenth century standardized hats into tricornes. The messenger on foot shows his hair tied back into a plait – an interesting military solution to long hair or periwigs, which were to make a big impact on fashion in the next century. (*Rijksmusum, Amsterdam*)

and archers, and some 400 horseguards glittering in gold and silver. To keep the nobility at court, spending money, most of the posts were quartered among four holders who had to serve for three months at a time. Thus Visconti could list Maximilian Antoine de Belleforière, the Duc d'Enghien and the Prince de Marsillac as grand masters of the wardrobe, a post often combined with that of grand huntsmen. Marsillac had been appointed in 1672, the eldest son of the Duc de La Rochefoucauld, when the previous incumbent the Marquis de Cessac had been found cheating at cards and was banished from court. The amount of attention which even ministers had to give to their appearance amazed Visconti. The Marquis de Louvois and the Marquis de Villeroi shut themselves up in a chamber for days to discuss the best position of a ribbon on a suit.[9]

The royal theatre could inspire fashions. The designer, 'dessinateur du cabinet du Roy', was Henri Gissey until his death in 1673, when he was succeeded by his pupil Jean Berain. A skirt Gissey created for the tragédie-ballet *Psyché* in 1671, composed by Molière and Corneille, became a fashionable sensation into 1673 for the decorative use of lace in three rows. Mantos were just coming into vogue that year too, often in Indian cloth. The most fashionable colour was of course flame, Louis XIV's favourite, as in flame-coloured satin mantos patterned with a little white. The distinctive feature of mantos was that they were loose and unboned, and not unlike the Indian gowns worn as dressing gowns. Both shared a kimono-like construction, and ladies loved

26 French School, 'Madame de Montespan with her Children by Louis XIV'.
The wildly extravagant marquise snatched the king from La Vallière in 1667, and her style was ostentation rather than good taste. Her tendency to plumpness was always a problem. On the far right in a riding habit is her elder son by the king, Louis Duc de Maine, not yet breeched, then come the daughters Françoise Marie and Louise Françoise, and the baby Louis Alexandre Comte de Toulouse. The last was born in 1678 which dates the painting to about 1680. (*Versailles; photograph Lauros-Giraudon*)

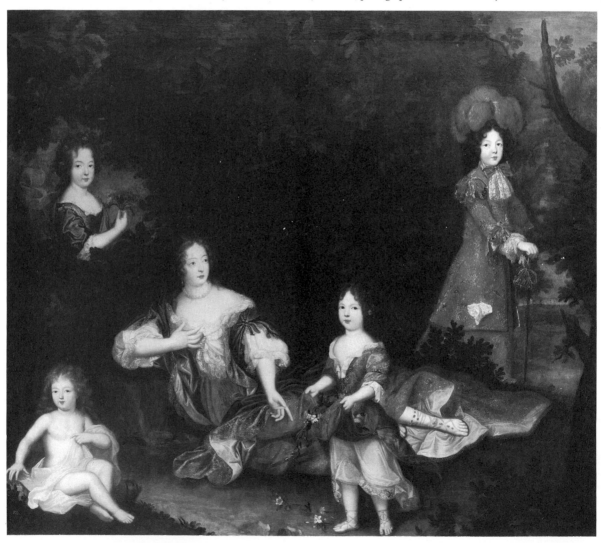

them as undress. At court, however, they had to wear full dress, with boned bodices.[20]

An act of royal hypocrisy came in 1675. Louis XIV asked Madame to Montespan to leave court for Easter; in other words he was giving up sex for the moment. She went to the mansion in the rue Vaugirard in Paris where the widow Scarron was raising her illegitimate children by the king.

One piece of gossip which intrigued Visconti was that the Marquise de Montespan lay naked on her bed every morning for two to three hours being anointed with perfumes and pomades. She wore so much scent that Louis XIV said it gave him a headache, to which she retorted that he smelt. The relationship was approaching a decline. The sort of clothes this mistress inspired were luxurious in the extreme: Madame de Sevigné wrote on 6 November 1676: 'Monsieur de Langlée has given Madame de Montespan a robe of gold on gold, re-embroidered with gold, with gold embroidery on top, and above a gold twisted and curled, mixed with a certain gold, which makes the most divine stuff which has ever been imagined.'

The chief sensation for 1676 were the transparents. These consisted of a dress in blue or gold brocade covered with a transparent dress in black or the finest English point lace, or else velvet chenille on a gossamer tissue. 'That', wrote the Marquise de Sevigné, 'composes a transparent, which is a black dress, or a dress all in gold or silver or colour, as you wish, and that is the fashion.'[21] It typified Louis XIV's requirement for luxurious style.

It was about this time that Louis XIV banned a particular colour, according to Madame de Montespan, although she did not give the date. The king had invaded the Netherlands in 1672 by crossing the Rhine, but the campaign was not going so well as he had expected. The Dutch flooded their fields and their new leader, William III Prince of Orange, still only in his twenties, was proving a resolute opponent. Peeved at this impertinence of opposing his will, Louis XIV banned orange – the fruit, the varnish, the colour in fabrics. All orange fabrics had to be redyed, and the prince of that name became unmentionable.[22]

The chief fashion news for 1678 was still the amount of gold and silver worn at court, either in cloth of gold and silver, or else on fabrics in the new colours of musk and brown, embroidered with gold and silver. There was even gold and silver embroidery on Naples laces, on silk, and on shaved velvet. For men the chief colours were grey coats or embroidered stuffs. At

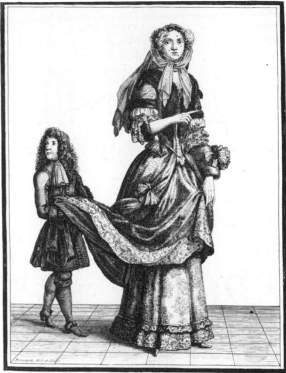

Dame en habit d'hyver.
Bien qu'elle fasse la Sucrée   Qu'elle est de malice fourée.
L'on juge à ce petit Sousris   Plus que de Martre ou petit gris.
Chez N. Bonnart, rue S.¹ Iacques, a l'Aigle. auec priuil.

27 Nicholas Bonnart, 'Lady in Winter Dress', c. 1678.
In the 1670s the Petite Académie began to allow the printing of huge numbers of fashion engravings to promote French style abroad, which were eagerly collected in England and Germany. This lady wears a fur tippet *à la palatine* which Elisabeth Charlotte had brought from Germany in 1671; it became a French fashion in 1676. The puffs have completely banished ringlets by now, and the line of the 1670s was lean after the bulbous 1660s. Embroidered fabrics were all the rage. (*Stadtmuseum, Munich*)

court however, embroidered coats were now reserved for the wearers of the *Juste-au-Corps à Brevet* (see page 61), yet coats in blue and red covered with French or Spanish point lace looked as good as embroidery. Tie a sash across the hips in gold or silver Spanish point lace, at the low-waist level, and the result was admirable. Add, of course, gold buttons, gold shoe buckles, gold ribbons, and gold-embroidered beaver hats, to achieve the glittering effect the king wanted to see on his courtiers. For ladies horse colour, mouse grey and pearl grey, covered with floral embroidery to imitate lace, were the new tones. Heavy satins with flowers in a raised surface like velvet carved into stamens of flowers were the latest luxury. Lace was so

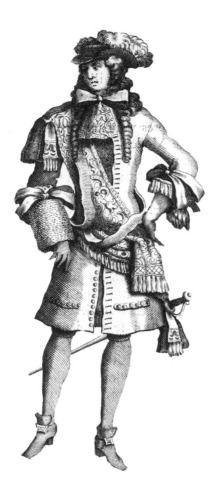

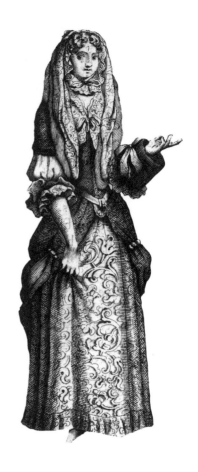

fashionable it led to the head being covered again, and eventually to the return of the married woman's cap. This fashion started by ladies wearing over the hair lengths of lace called *cornetes* (pinners in England). A fine lace such as the Queen's point was best, as French point was too thick, and the fashion was to wear two layers. The *cornete* hung down on either side of the face, but the *petite cornete* was fastened under the chin by a ribbon bow. If a third layer was added, it was usually decorated with casual knots. The manto was increasingly popular for informal occasions, and the best colour for 1678 was musk-coloured satin embroidered with linen grey and violet, worn over a heavy satin petticoat in off white, embroidered with blue and violet or musk. The chief characteristic of the silhouette throughout this decade was its increasing slimness, deflating the large sleeves, wide skirts and coats of the 1660s into a tighter line.

28 'Cavalier in Winter Dress', 1678, from *Le Nouveau Mercure Galant*.
The first appearance of fashion engravings in a monthly magazine. The *Mercure Galant* was revived in 1677 to be another form of propaganda for the Crown. The style promoted, however, is the English type of suit with the coat and vest to the knee, now so established that the French were regarding it as theirs. It shows the leaner line of that decade with longer sleeves and small hats. There is one bow of ribbon at the cravat, which had begun to oust wide collars in the late 1660s. (*The British Library*)

29 'Lady in Winter Attire' 1678, from *Le Nouveau Mercure Galant*.
The fashion for lace brought back womens' caps in the form of pinners or *cornetes*, which were both headscarves and caps tied under under the chin. The low waistline typified the period, producing the long effect that was part of the lean ideal. The skirt appears to have an embossed pattern.

Monsieur Charlier of the rue de la Coutellerie in Paris, at the Golden Hoop, had been appointed royal silk mercer in 1672, and his satins, damask, cloth of gold and silks clothed the king and his household thereafter. His establishment was the place to find the most fabulous fabrics imaginable. For cloth one had to go to Sieur Gaultier who sold the greys for men's suits and coats.[23]

In 1679 the Duchesse d'Orléans, Elisabeth Charlotte, received a visit from her youngest paternal aunt, Sophia Duchess of Hanover, mother of Britain's future King George I. As a Protestant she could not receive full formalities at this Catholic court, but as Louis XIV wanted everybody to see his glory, she could appear *incognito* by wearing a black sash and using a lesser title, as Madame d'Osnabrück. Sophia recorded 'As Monsieur did not wish to be ashamed of anyone he was to introduce at court, he insisted on helping to choose the stuffs which we were to wear on so great an occasion.' Accordingly Aunt Sophia had to endure the attentions of French dressmakers and

30 Jan van Kessel, 'A Spanish Family in a Garden', 1680. The Spanish attempted to remain distinct, but signs of a collapse were creeping in. While the men have mostly the sober Spanish court style with the golilla collar, the boys have Anglo-French suits. The women wear their hair down in the Spanish way, and the bulbous bottom sleeve also seems local. The French court was determined to subjugate all foreign styles, but particularly the Spanish style. (*Museo del Prado, Madrid*)

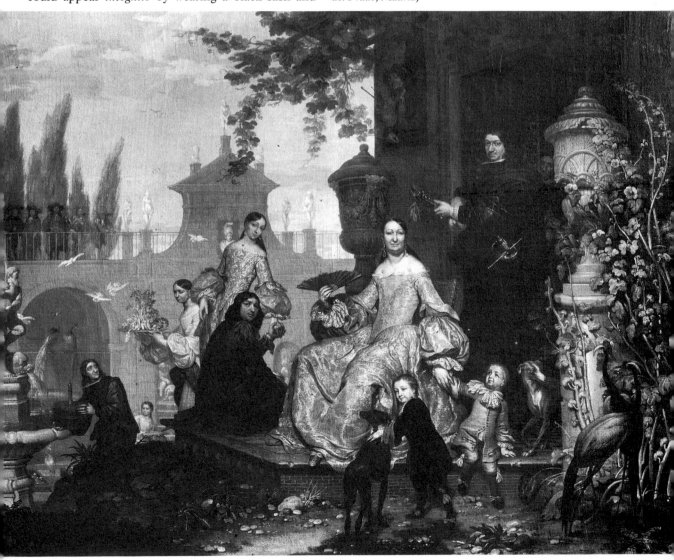

tailors who dressed her, and patched her face into *le style français*. She was in time to see the proxy wedding of Monsieur's eldest daughter Marie Louise to Carlos II of Spain. Monsieur Philippe was all excitement and took her into a boudoir at Fontainebleau to see the coat he was having embroidered with diamonds for the occasion. When Sophia called on her niece late at night she found them undressed:

I found her in a dressing gown, also Monsieur, who wore a nightcap, tied with flame coloured ribbons, was arranging some jewels for Madame, himself and his two daughters. He was much confused at being seen in this guise, and turned his head from side to side, but I quite put him at ease, by helping him with the jewels, and making a bow for his hat, with which he seemed much pleased. After completing a work of such importance, I could sleep in peace.

The 'two daughters' refers to the two Monsieur had had by his first wife Henriette Anne. He now had two more children by Elisabeth Charlotte, a son Philippe Duc de Chartres born in 1674, and the baby Elisabeth Charlotte. At the marriage service the king's eye was mostly on the young Mademoiselle de Fontanges while the Marquise de Montespan sulked in undress. 'The Queen, was, I thought, much incommoded by her dress, for, notwithstanding the extreme heat, her skirt was covered with embroidery heavier than that which is put on horses' trappings.' The weight of French court embroidery was one of Madame Elisabeth Charlotte's complaints as well. Her aunt found the Dauphin uninteresting, and thought the Prince de Conti looked 'actually common', for all his cloak was covered with diamonds. Monsieur later, seizing a candle, proceeded to treat the Queen Marie Thérèse as a living exhibit while he walked round her, pointing out the best jewels in the royal collection. Sophia declined to kiss the queen's skirt, being a sovereign lady, and refused the offer of a stool, for the empress in Vienna, although a Catholic, had granted her family an armchair. Madame Martin was still the top hair stylist and did Marie Louise's hair for her,

while the new queen of Spain applied rouge, which all the Spanish princesses wore.[24]

Not surprisingly as soon as Marie Louise reached Spain she was stripped of all French finery. There was no love for Louis XIV there after he had occupied the Spanish Netherlands. The wife of the French ambassador, the Marquise de Villars, wrote from Madrid on 30 November 1679 that Marie Louise had greeted the king in a beautiful French dress and an astonishing amount of precious stones, but the very next day she was put into a Spanish dress which the king much preferred. La Martin's hairstyles were undone for the simple Spanish look with the hair brushed across the forehead, and spread out on the shoulders.[25]

On her way back to Hanover, Sophia visited her sick niece the Duchesse d'Enghien and found her in 'a gold brocade sacque tied all the way down with flame-coloured ribbon, which had, as I thought, a very startling effect'. Even so, she had been impressed by the dazzling finery she had seen at Versailles, Fontainebleau, and Monsieur Philippe's residence at St Cloud. The amount of wealth worn on the backs of the French court was staggering – all that cloth of gold and silver smothered with diamonds and other jewels. Accordingly, Sophia arranged for Abbé Ballati to be her agent in Paris, whenever she had special events in her calendar, such as the marriages of her children and subsequently of grandchildren. This set a pattern which other German princes followed. The Marquise de Montespan had been most scornful the first time she saw a German prince visit Louis XIV, from Würtemburg; he wore an old-fashioned doublet with copper buttons, no periwig, no ribbons or lace, and no gold buckles on his shoes which were fastened with red leather bows. The Germans, however, could be excused for looking dowdy when they had just endured the Thirty Years War, and Louis XIV was going to involve them in even more wars. The French Impact was two-edged.

TWO

The Textile War

The man who had to finance Louis XIV's glory, after the ousting of Nicolas Fouquet, was Colbert. As early as 1648 Colbert had shown his economic approach 'by changing the fine Silver Edgings that were fitted to the Ribbons with which the Habits of the Hundred Switzers were adorn'd, to counterfeit Lace'[1]. It was Fouquet who recommended Colbert to Cardinal Mazarin when he was in exile and needed someone in Paris to manage his financial affairs. The careful Colbert so impressed the cardinal that he gave him increasing responsibility, and in 1653 Colbert sent the cardinal an outline of his thoughts for future policy:

We must re-establish or create all industries, even luxury industries; a system of protection must be established by means of a customs tariff; trade and traders must be organized into guilds; financial hindrances which burden the people must be lightened; transport of commodities by sea and land must be restored; colonies must be developed and commercially bound to France; all barriers between France and India must be broken down; the Navy must be strengthened in order to afford protection to merchant ships.[2]

Once Colbert was appointed to run the national finances he put this policy into practice. He began by recouping for the Crown the excessive profits that its officials had creamed off since 1635. This caused panic in Paris and some rich men fled abroad. Colbert established the Chambre de Justice, which proceeded to fine 4,000 financiers for their profiteering and recouped 100 million livres for the Crown. Kings like that sort of minister. Colbert abolished the hereditary nature of many financial posts, forced officials to keep proper accounts, and put the tax-farm system out to bids. He even taught Louis XIV to do accounts, not that this had much impact on his mania for glory. Still, if the king wanted splendour, Colbert would ensure that the money involved would remain inside France.[3]

Colbert was a firm believer in sumptuary law, and wrote to the king:

We daily see Laws last but a little time, and are frequently broken as soon as made. *Your Majesty* must therefore lay a Tax upon all those that wear Clothes beyond their Quality, and you must by an Edict declare who may wear Gold and Silver, who Silk, and so downwards; and that they who ought not to wear Gold or Silver, and yet presume to do it, shall pay so much; and they that wear Silk, or any other forbidden Stuff, so much.

He suggested fines starting at one crown.[4]

The *Declaration du Roy* issued on 30 June 1661 stated 'We wish Our subjects to wear French trimmings and lace, not foreign.' Decoration on clothes should not be more than two fingers high, and not exceed 40 sols in cost. Such decoration might be applied to clothes, but no additional finery was allowed in between. Men might only have lace or trimmings around the collar, on the hem of a cloak, down the sides of canons and breeches, on the seams of sleeves, around the head of a sleeve, down the centre back seam, around the edge of basques, and down the buttons front and around the buttonholes. Women might only wear lace or trimmings around the hem of the petticoat and down the front of gowns and skirts, and around basques and on bodices. Merchants who sold foreign lace and trimming would be fined 1,500 livres. Further restrictions were issued in 1664, and the *Declaration du Roy* was renewed on 23 November 1667, again banning the wearing of foreign lace and ornamentation. On 17 March 1668 Venetian point lace and Genoese lace were banned.

There were geographical problems in trying to set up industries in France. An attempt to reproduce London serge at Gournay failed because French wool was so inferior to English, and French sheep much smaller than the Cotswold type with its long fleece that was the delight of weavers. English calfskin could not be imitated in France, so Louis XIV wore English,

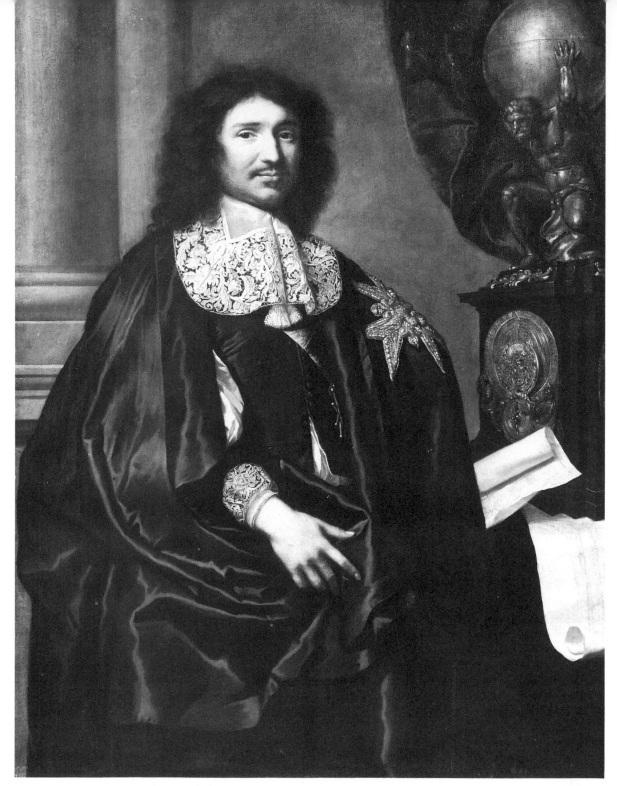

31 Claude LeFebvre, 'Jean Baptiste Colbert'.
The controller general of finances, the superintendent of buildings and the minister for the Navy was popularly known as the North Wind. A strong believer in protectionism, he erected barriers against foreign products but sought to flood foreign markets with French goods. To achieve this he needed to import foreign experts and English wool. Thus the European reaction against Louis XIV and France was a mixture of economic as well as national feeling. (*Versailles, cliché des Musées Nationaux*)

because French cattle were inferior. River water varied from region to region so not every town could have a dye works. To improve matters Colbert imported foreign experts from across Europe: Dutch and Flemish weavers and clothmakers; English goldsmiths, leathermen and stocking makers; Italian lacemakers; German metalworkers; Spanish leatherworkers, hatters and weavers; tarmakers from Scandinavia and leather men from Russia. All such countries attempted to restrict this loss of expertise, and Venice even poisoned two Venetians who worked at the mirror factory in Paris. In 1665 Colbert persuaded the Protestant manufacturer Josse van Robais of Zeeland to move to Abbéville with 50 Dutch weavers, with no duty to pay on his looms, and freedom from French guild restrictions. By 1680 Robais had increased to 80 looms, producing 1,600 pieces of cloth a year, and employed 1,690 people. This firm continued in France until the Revolution. Two other Dutch Protestants were invited to Elbeuf to improve the local white cloth, a rough type used for peasants' overcoats. They created *drap d'Elbeuf* as a finer version, and by 1693 the town had 300 looms and 8,000 workers producing 9 to 10,000 pieces a year. The Dutch experts left, however, after Revocation of the Edict of Nantes in 1685 cancelled all Protestant rights; Elbeuf began to decline.

The English James Fournier was granted letters patent on 27 July 1663 to open an English silk stocking factory at the Château de Madrid in Paris. The stockings were knitted on a frame, unlike woollen stockings which had to be knitted by hand, and the French were keen to learn the English technique. By 1669 Colbert claimed 32 French towns could produce English-type silk stockings. This hit the English producers very hard. Colbert invited 38 French towns to produce Venetian lace, having banned the original, but this met with mixed success. Alençon thrived, and Auxerre failed.

In 1664 the importation of foreign tapestries was banned to help the French tapestry weavers at Gobelins. Colbert purchased the building, put up the royal coat of arms and the title *manufacture royale*, and appointed Le Brun as director. This was to be the leading works to decorate Versailles and in 1667 Louis XIV issued an edict which allowed Gobelins to specialize in luxury products for the palace – sculptures, candelebras, vases, tapestries and locks. The staff included the engravers Le Clerc and Le Pautre to produce prints of court fashion, and this encouraged other engravers to follow suit. From the 1670s French fashion plates began to spread across Europe, advertising the superiority of French taste. Samuel Pepys collected them and so did German princes.[5]

To clothe the court, regulations were issued for the silk trade in Lyons in 1667, and in Paris in 1669. Lyons, for example, was allowed to make 13 classifications of stuffs: cloth of gold and silver, brocades, satins, damasks and velvets; fine silks without gold or silver; striped stuffs, dappled and wide-striped fabrics; lustrous black taffeta, ordinary taffeta, velvet and satin; flat woven stuffs; mixed materials with goathair, cotton and wool as in camlets, and moirés (mohair); imitation gold and silver fabrics; light materials such as gauze, silk tissue, and crêpe.[6] Lyons silk production soared to meet the court's requirements for luxury. In 1621 there were 1,648 looms, in 1660 3,296, and in 1720 5,067, producing a variety of figured silks and bullion-flowered brocades. Apprenticeships were set for five years, and in 1678 the minimum age for entry was 13. A silk weaver's widow could continue his trade with his existing apprentices, but she could not take on new ones.

The biggest French fabric export was linen grown and made in Picardy, Normandy and Brittany. The Crown granted monopolies so that Rheims and Le Mans specialized in muslin, Picardy and Champagne made coarse cloth, and Languedoc a slightly better cloth, while Amiens was known for mixed cloth. Cloth and linen were produced as piece work by country weavers who were peasants trying to earn a little extra, hence the need to import Dutch professionals to set up manufactories. France was also behind in trading overseas, for England had the East India Company which received its charter from Elizabeth I in 1600, and the Dutch East India Company was started in 1602. To compete Colbert set up a whole range of companies. In 1664 he founded the French East India Company and the French West India Company; in 1665 the French North African Company followed. 1669 saw the French Company of the North established to trade in the Baltic, 1670 the French Levant Company founded. The French Senegal Company arrived in 1673, the French Hudson Bay Company in 1682, the French China Company in 1698, and the French Guinea Company in 1701. The battle was on, for the trade of the Indies in particular.

Cardinal Mazarin had started a protective tariff barrier over 1644–54 when he increased the duties on Dutch and Flemish camlet and English cloth fivefold. Colbert continued this by increasing the tariff on

Dutch goods even higher in 1664, with the result that the Dutch in 1670 started to boycott French products.[7] England reacted by banning foreign bone-lace, cut work, embroidery, fringe, band-strings, buttons and needlework in 1662 under the statute Caroli II c. 13. That same year Caroli II c. 18 banned the export of sheeps' wool. The one item France required to improve its own cloth was English wool. The English of course wanted to keep the work of weaving into cloth in their country, and they kept pressurizing Charles II to take firm action. Unfortunately they faced an evasive monarch who was very pro-French and from 1670 actually in the pay of the French government, so a total ban on French trade did not appear. To help the wool industry the British government decided to reduce the import of French linen by introducing in 1666 an 'Act for burying in woollen only'. From now on all shrouds had to be in wool not linen. The Act was not strong enough, so in 1677 it was replaced by one which required that from 1 August 1678

no corps of any person shall be buried in any shirt, shift, sheet, or shroud, of any thing whatsoever made or mingled with flax, hemp, silk, hair, gold or silver, or in any stuff or thing, other than what is made of sheeps wool only, or be put in any coffin lined or faced with any sort of cloth or stuff, or any other thing whatsoever, that is made of any material but sheeps wool only.

The clergy had to keep a register of materials used in burials, and fines were set at £5. An oath that a deceased person had been buried in wool had to be taken before a Justice of the Peace. In 1680 this was modified to empower mayors and city bailiffs to administer the oath, as not everybody had a JP in the vicinity.

Since 1663 Parliament had been saying there ought to be a ban on imported clothes, and on 26 October 1665/6 Lord Arlington wrote to the Lord Mayor of London:

The King, considering that vast sums are yearly exported for foreign manufacturers, whilst both in France and Holland, vigorous ways are used to discourage English manufacturers, has resolved that, after the mourning for the King of Spain is over [Philip IV], he will wear nothing, inside or out, that is not English manufacture, except linen and calicoes. The Queen will do the same, and whole Court is enjoined to follow their example. Wishes the London shopkeepers to know this, that they may not send abroad for laces, silks, stuff &c.[8]

The following year Charles II launched the long English vest and the English three-piece suit, but a national fashion and asking people not to wear foreign clothes were gestures, not compulsion.

Colbert was out to exclude English cloth completely, and raised the duty twice to 25 and 50 per cent, and he cancelled the standing order for English grey to clothe the French infantry. Bedford Whiting wrote to Secretary Williamson on 31 December 1670:

They are subtle enough yet to let our wools come in free, without which they cannot make all their new fashioned stuffs, which makes them the more presume to prohibit our manufactures.

Whereas we usually furnished the French, for clothing their soldiers with a coarse sort of light grey cloth, Colbert obliged all the infantry to be clothed with a cloth called Serge de Berry, made about Rouen; it is tolerably good for clothing, but it is not to be made without English wool, and unless it came to hanging for wool stealing – as indeed all thieves ought, and especially such notorious thieves as rob a whole kingdom – in time we shall lose the reputation of our fabrics.

Strangers I find are more thrifty than we are; they can work cheaper than we, and they have many pleasing inventions, which we are not addicted to, and by making so many new fabrics, the French fabrics are in greater estimation than many of ours. There are able heads in England to consult on matters of trade, but I fear we are not so diligent as our neighbours.[9]

It was not a lack of diligence, however, which caused the English government not to place huge tariffs on French textiles. It was in 1670 that Charles II accepted the bribe from Louis XIV, so he was in the pay of the enemy. A great clamour arose to negotiate a new trade treaty with France. The gentlemen, MPs and JPs of Wiltshire petitioned the government that the export of their undyed white pack cloth be not prohibited, for it employed 30,000 people. The clothiers of Berkshire, Worcester, Stafford, Devon, Oxford, Suffolk, Coventry and Kent argued that the work of finishing and dyeing cloth should stay in England. The clothworkers and dyers of London supported this view, and the woad merchants said there was such a decline in dyeing at home that they would have to discontinue planting woad. The government replied that a limited export of undyed wool was beneficial; in other words, Charles II would not annoy the French. He made another gesture by wearing mixed cloths of silk and wool in the summer of 1676, which helped the sales of mixed cloths, but offered no help to pure cloth. Faced with Colbert's tariffs the export of cloth fell from 90,000 pieces to

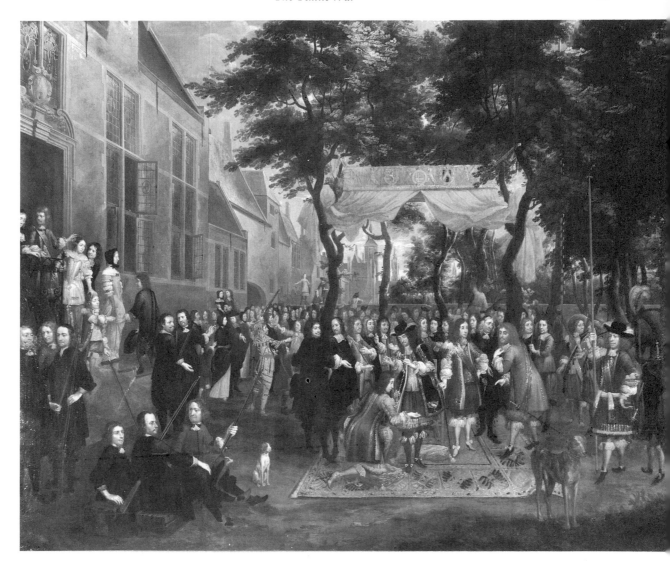

20,000 by 1677, and the French were also encroaching on England's old markets in the Netherlands and Germany.[10]

The trade imbalance was such that in 1674 France bought English silk and linen of the value of £85,000, but England imported £800,000 worth of French silk and linen. Add to this French wine and brandy, lace and embroidery, and the deficit between the two was £1,000,000. It was only slightly better in 1676 according to the notes of secretary Williamson of the Committee of Trade: England exported £171,000 to France of which £63,000 was woollen goods, but she imported French linen worth £507,000, French silks worth £300,000, and French wine and brandy worth £200,000.[11]

32 J. Meunincxhove, 'Charles II and James Duke of York in the Gardens of the Guild of Sainte Barbe', s.d. 1671. Charles II, who had launched the English suit, was ordered by his sister Henriette Anne to give it up, as required by Louis XIV. This Flemish painting suggests that he obeyed. Charles II on the carpet is depicted entirely in the French style with a short coat, petticoat breeches and a short vest. Charles II would do nothing to risk his French 'subsidy', despite the huge petitions from English merchants for him to act against Colbert's trade barriers. The visit depicted had taken place in 1656, but was not recorded until 1671 in the dress of the later date. Note the medieval fool whom courts still maintained. (*Musée Groeninge, Bruges, copyright ACL Brussels*)

Sir George Downing said in 1676 that the king and queen ought to wear only English silk and English lace, so clearly Charles II was not honouring his promise of 1665/6, which he had repeated in 1673 and 1675. In May 1673 Charles received a petition:

The Weavers' Company of London to the King and Privy Council. Petition on behalf of themselves and all other English weavers stating the great discouragement of the petitionees by the frequent importations of foreign wrought silks, ribbons, laces &c., by which some thousands of them have been forced to forsake their callings, and that though during the past eight years the consumption of such commodities has greatly increased not one fourth of the handicraftsmen have been or are now employed as heretofore.

The Company called for a ban on imported items, mainly French. Charles II responded:

Declaration of the King in Council in pursuance of the address of Parliament and the application of the Weavers' Company, that he has resolved henceforth to wear none but English manufactures, except linen and calico and has ordered the Master of the Great Wardrobe to buy none other for this use, and the Lord High Chamberlain not to permit any persons to come into the presence wearing foreign manufactures, also that the Lord Treasurer give orders for seizing all foreign goods imported contrary to the law, the King's moiety thereof to be burnt.[12]

How the Lord High Chamberlain was to distinguish foreign clothes and fabric was not defined. It was another of Charles II's high-sounding gestures, which did not put a tariff of 25 or 50 per cent on French silks. He made a similar response in July 1675 after being appealed to about the imports of French lace.

Memorandum that his Majesty, having declared that day in Council that he would not wear any foreign points or laces after his return to Whitehall, likewise ordered that after Michaelmas next none of his subjects wear any such points or laces, and the Lord Chamberlain of the Household is not to permit any of his subjects wearing such points or laces to appear in his Majesty's presence.[13]

Yet the wearing of foreign lace had been banned back in 1662, so by promising to give it up in 1675, Charles II showed that he had broken his own government's law frequently. Once more he declined to erect a trade barrier against France, being in French pay. The Act of 1662 was not renewed or extended with greater powers, and the statement of 1675 that his subjects were not to wear foreign lace did not require the magistracy to enforce it or establish a system of fines. Accordingly, as Charles II

well knew, his statement would soon be forgotten. No matter how much action Colbert took against English products, Charles II would not endanger his own French subsidy.

There was simply no equivalent of Colbert in England. He was the Chancellor of the Exchequer, the Minister for Economic Development, and the Minister for the Navy combined in one. It took the Glorious Revolution of 1688 to oust the Catholic Stuarts from the British thrones and replace them with the Protestant Mary II and her Dutch husband William of Orange, the determined enemy of Louis XIV and France. In 1689 came the declaration that English wool merchants and weavers longed to hear – a complete ban on trade with France. The French wine and brandy industry suffered greatly as a result, and the French woollen cloth industry was desperate. It could not continue without English wool, so it offered a high price for smuggled wool and a local industry in smuggling began to thrive in Romney Marshes: English wool for French brandy. The ban lasted until 1717, and it was by force of arms that England, Denmark and Norway obliged Louis XIV to reduce French tariffs against their good, in 1711.

To encourage English trade William and Mary set up in 1690 the King and Queen's Corporation for Linen Manufacture to introduce new techniques, by granting letters patent to Nicholas Dupin and Henry Million. In 1692 they approved the grant of letters patent to Paul Cloudesley, William Sherrard and Peter Duclew for a new invention for making black lustring and dressed silks. In 1694 Francis Pousset received letters patent for his prepared crépes, and that year Peter Oliver was similarly licensed to produce his engine for beautifying linen cloth, silks and calicoes by glazing. A patent for calico printing had been granted to John Pons and David Cossart in 1693 who claimed that their prints resisted washing, boiling and bleaching. In 1695 Ralph Law was empowered to proceed with his scheme for dyeing cloth on one side only. In Ireland William Sutton, George Hagar, and Edmund Buckridge were granted letters patent for their waterproofing method for linen, wool, silk and leather. The new government waged war against France on the battlefield, and encouraged textile development at home. In 1693 Mary II commanded the Attorney General to prosecute wool smugglers and stealers with severity for they were breaking the law by trading with France and they were corresponding with the enemy. In 1689 William and Mary invited French Protestant refugees, the Huguenots to take refuge in England, and the French names mentioned above reflect this influx of talent.[14]

Jean Baptiste Colbert died in 1683, having dedicated himself to making France self-reliant in as many industries as possible. He might well have queried the wisdom of forcing French Protestants to abjure their faith or flee, for it hit the very industries he had tried to build up. But Louis XIV was now approaching middle age and had begun to worry about his sinful past. The one act which would make the Catholic Church forgive him everything would be to revoke his grandfather's Edict of Nantes and extinguish the Reformed Church in France. Between 1661 and 1679 there had been 12 restrictions on Protestant life; between 1679 and 1685 this was increased to 85. They were banned from all offices, and could not be judges, lawyers, bailiffs, booksellers, printers, doctors or secretaries. From 1675 to 1685 300 Protestant churches were demolished. Only one Protestant school teacher was allowed per town, regardless of the number of Protestant children, to force them to use Catholic schools. In 1680 the notorious *Dragonnades* began, the billeting of royal dragoons on Protestant families, at their own expense. They had orders to behave badly, and proceeded to beat, torture, rob, rape, and burn their hosts. The atrocities became so bad that cardinals Le Camus of Grenoble and de Coislin of Orléans ordered the dragoons to leave their dioceses. Louis XIV was informed that all the Protestants in France had accepted conversion to Catholicism, and could claim that the Edict of Nantes was no longer necessary, so he revoked it in 1685. Protestant pastors were given two weeks to leave the country; nobody else was free to go, but approximately a quarter of a million French Protestants, the Huguenots, escaped to the Netherlands, England, Switzerland, Germany and Scandinavia. Louis XIV lost 600 army officers including a marshall of France, Schomberg, and the diplomat the Marquis de Ruvigny; they all offered their services to William of Orange. When Louis XIV sent the exiled James II to attack Britain in Ireland, he was defeated by an Anglo-Dutch army which contained four regiments of French Huguenots.[15]

The English silk industry benefited because many of the French refugees were weavers who established themselves in Spitalfields in London and were accepted into the English Weavers' Company. Mary II and William III, joint rulers, imitated Colbert's royal manufactories by licensing the Royal Lustring Company in 1692 which was run by the Frenchmen Louis Gervais, Peter Le Keux and Hilary Reneu. James Leman became a celebrated designer and manufacturer of silks, Monceaux, Mariscot and Lanson were known for figured silks, and Christopher Baudoin became the most famous silk designer in England, in the early 1700s. The most famous French Huguenot name in British textiles, Courtauld, belonged to a family who fled to London as goldsmiths and pursued that trade into the 1780s, when marriage with the Ogiers of Spitalfields turned their interest into silks and crêpes; by 1898 this had led to the invention of artificial silks and rayons. Colbert must have spun in his grave. He had devoted so much attention to importing foreign experts to increase the quality of French products, and to train French specialists, but Louis XIV had driven many of those specialists abroad and England and the Netherlands were reaping the benefit! They were not all saints, for the former Lyons silk merchant Seignoret was found guilty of smuggling in French lustring silks in 1698 and fined £10,000, but the majority of the immigrants subscribed to the Protestant Work Ethic and set up many businesses, from design to wine.[16]

In their invitation to French Huguenots William and Mary promised help:

By the King and Queen,
A DECLARATION
For the Encouraging of French *Protestants to Transport themselves into this Kingdom*
Whereas it hath pleased Almighty God to Deliver Our Realm of *England* and the Subjects thereof, from the Persecution lately threatening them for their Religion, and from the Oppression and Destruction which the Subversion of the Laws, and the Arbitrary Exercise of Power and Dominion over them had very near introduced; We find in Our Subjects a True and Just Sense hereof, and of the Miseries and Oppressions the *French* Protestants lye under; For their Relief, and to Encourage them that shall be willing to Transport themselves, their Families and Estates, into this Our Kingdom, We do hereby Declare, That all *French* Protestants that shall seek refuge in, and Transport themselves into this Our Kingdom, shall not only have Our Royal Protection for themselves, Families, and Estates within this Our Realm, But We will also do Our Endeavour in all reasonable Ways and Means so to Support, Aid and Assist them in their several Trades and Ways of Livelyhood, as that their living and being in this Realm may be comfortable and easie to them.
Given at Our Court at Whitehall *this Twenty fifth Day of* April, 1689, *In the First Year of Our Reign.*
God Save the King and Queen.

They kept this promise establishing the royal companies, by granting letters patent to French experts and innovators, and by giving money through the Civil List. Parliament made an annual grant to French Protestant churches, French pastors and French refugees and their descendants right through the eighteenth century. Two soup kitchens in Soho and Spitalfields were set up for the poorest and continued to help them for a century.

Soho was the centre for fashionable shops, and as late as 1738 French was still spoken there by Huguenot families. Ralph Duke of Montagu, Master of the Wardrobe to William III, engaged many refugee craftsmen, and patronized the French tailor Joseph Boucher in London. Huguenots worked on the completion of Hampton Court Palace and on Montagu's own house. Daniel Marot was appointed architect to William III, Jean Tijou the ironsmith designed and made the gates for Hampton Court Palace, and the Huguenot upholsterer François Lapierre provided the crimson silk velvet and Chinese silk damask state bed. The royal patronage could hardly have been more generous in English circumstances, although the monarchs could not rival Louis XIV in the scale of building and decoration, for their powers were now limited by Parliament. Louis XIV thought the English would never stomach a Dutch king, but overlooked the fact that William's wife and mother were British. The joint monarchy was welcomed, and kept its promises.[17] William III knew from experience that the only way to persuade Louis XIV to reduce his protective barrier against foreign goods was on the battlefield. As Prince of Orange he had managed to obtain a reduction in the tariffs on Dutch goods when he beat Louis XIV's attempt to take over the Netherlands. In 1678 the Treaty of Nijmegen obliged Louis XIV to put the tariffs down to the rate of 1664. As king of the United Kingdoms William applied the same policy by seeking to block Louis's colonial ambitions abroad, and organizing confederations against him in Europe. Colbert had built up a magnificent navy to win France colonies, but the Anglo-Dutch fleet burnt it at La Hogue in 1692 right in front of Louis XIV's eyes. All the golden splendour of the carved sterns, the most elaborate in any navy, proved to be no more than show. In 1690 William III had observed that Lord Marlborough was most suitable for great commands. After William's death in 1702 his sister-in-law Queen Anne gave Marlborough his opportunity to halt the invincible French army, and once again this proved

the only way to obtain a reduction in the tariffs on British products in 1711. Thus the protective wall against imports erected by Mazarin and Colbert was literally battered down by France's chief rivals. The attempts of the French East India Company to dominate India were beaten by the British East India Company in the years to come, and France would lose Canada. Colbert's colonial schemes were reduced to a few islands.

Inside France Colbert influenced the construction of clothes. In 1655 the Master Merchant Tailors' guild and the guild of Doublet (*pour point*) Makers united to create the Master Merchant Tailors Doubleters. Their new statutes were approved by the procurator general at the Châtelet on 22 May 1660, and they received letters patent granting them the sole right to make tailored clothes. Apprenticeships were set at three years. Colbert was a firm believer in industry being organized, so in 1675 he set out to found a system for sewing women. The standard must be raised to increase the reputation of French clothes, so an apprenticeship scheme was established as for tailors, with three years for the course. Girls could qualify in cutting and dressmaking and could graduate as a *couturière*, or cutter/seamstress. They could operate in four categories. The *couturière en habit* made women's clothes, the *couturière en corps d'enfant* made children's clothes, the *couturière en linge* made linen underwear, and the *couturière en garniture* specialized in the garnishing or trimmings. This pattern was soon being copied abroad, and by the 1680s professional dressmakers were beginning to oust ladies' tailors in Britain.[18]

To some extent defeats in the battlefield could be compensated for by publicity from the royal controlled Press. It was important to remind Europe of the glamour and glory of the French court. The sort of propaganda Louis XIV liked to hear was penned by the royal historiographer Boileau-Despréaux:

Versailles. Epistle VIII to the King.
In that sweet Dwelling, full of noble Charms,
The Hero shines as glorious in Arms,
Thou bear'st alone the Crown's increasing weight,
And art the only Atlas of the State.
Arts thou hast cherish'd, and with Hands profuse
Rewarded and Inrich'd the Critic Muse,
Thou ev'n to Satire dost thy Grace extend;
What Monarch was to Truth so much a Friend?[19]

It would be closer to the truth to observe that the arts were only allowed to glorify the king, and satire could

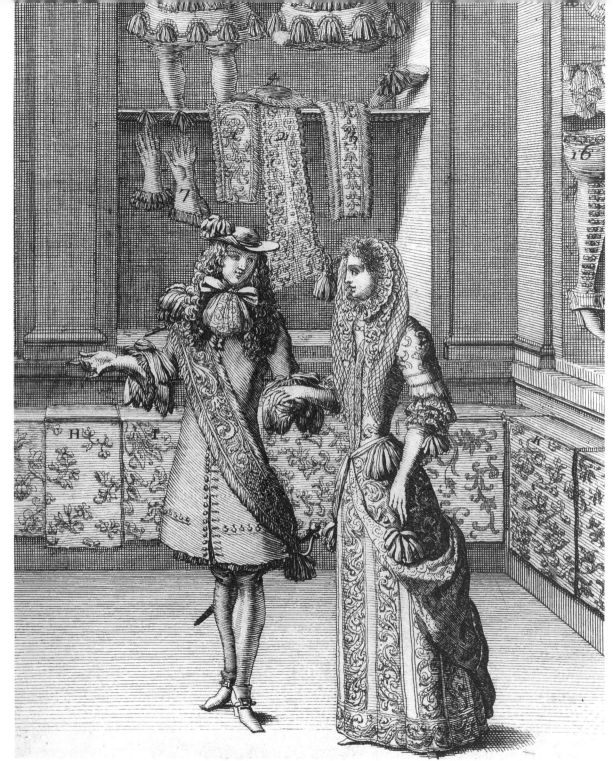

33 'Interior of a French Fabric and Dress Shop', from
Le Nouveau Mercure Galant, 1678.

The French silk industry swept to widespread success under Colbert's protection and Louis XIV's demands for luxurious fabrics, which were restricted by law to the upper class. Floral patterns dominated in the 1660s and 1670s but the woman's petticoat shows a few stripes which were to be the major design in the 1680s. The petticoat breeches on sale show how Louis XIV's fondness for them kept them going in France, but they were out-of-date as far as England and the Netherlands were concerned. The use of fringes on the baldrics and gloves was about to increase. (*Kunstbibliothek Charlottenburg Palace, Berlin, Proussischer Kulturbesitz*) mock the bourgeoisie but not the monarchy. In 1677 Sieur Blageart revived the monthly magazine *Le Mercure Galant* and renamed it *Le Nouveau Mercure Galant*. It was under the control of the royal censors from the start, and there may have been some government finance behind the publication, for it became the court journal. To the format of fashionable news, stories, latest songs, were added long celebrations of royal events, lengthy descriptions of royal magnificence, and lavish panegyrics on the sovereign's wisdom and splendour, and the invincibility of his armies. The magazine was turned into a stylish propaganda instrument for the superiority of the French court and culture. Month after month *Le Nouveau Mercure Galant* poured out detailed descriptions of royal balls, theatricals, masquerades, ballets, entries, reviews and firework festivals. If Louis XIV had begun to suffer some reversals in the battlefield, he did not intend to lose the propaganda war.

France also tried to evade the ban on trade with Britain by offering high prices for English raw wool smuggled out from the south coast. The wool factor John Haynes was appointed a commissioner in 1698 to supervise the ban on exports, but reported that the job was impossible. There was so much corruption among Army officers and local magistrates in Kent that few smugglers were caught and fined. Some people in high places had their fingers in the illegal trade, for the royal yacht *Isabella* was found to have raw wool hidden under the cabin bunks. The attorney general intervened, and nobody was prosecuted. Haynes wanted to see a government system of inspectors with their own ships to patrol the coast, but the government was too busy with the war against Louis XIV. Haynes was not in favour of a total ban on exporting raw wool, for Turkey sent raw silk and cotton into Britain, and Russia sent leather, hemp and fur. In both cases this provided work for English weavers, leather dressers and furriers, which would balance the loss of work involved in selling them raw wool. France however, and to some extent Spain and the Netherlands, demanded English raw wool to blend with their inferior native wools to improve the quality and double the quantity of their cloth production, to the detriment of British weavers who they did not help by sending raw silk or cotton to weave in return.[20]

A new threat to European textiles in general arose, because the successful English and Dutch East India Companies, which Colbert copied, all brought back great quantities of oriental fabrics. France took protective measures published on 26 October 1686. Too much East Indian printed calico, painted calico, and Indian and Chinese silks and flowered silks patterned with gold and silver, was being imported. The painting and printing of calico inside France was ordered to stop, the blocks must be burned, and a fine of 3,000 livres was established for any breach. Silk merchants might sell their existing stocks of oriental silks up to the end of December 1687, but thereafter all such stock in warehouses was to be burned. Here too the fine was set at 3,000 livres.[21] The textile war was entering a new dimension; no longer merely a European competition, it was becoming one which also involved the East.

THREE

Court Dress and Masquerades

It was in 1661 that Louis XIV first gave some thought to founding an official court dress restricted to a select few men, as one of the prizes to dangle before the aristocracy if it resided at court under the king's eye. According to the Abbé de Dangeau only 29 names were drawn up at that stage but in 1664/5 the number was set at 50. This privileged group was to have a special coat, for coats were the latest fashion in the early 1660s, with the right to wear ornamentation which sumptuary law banned for lesser beings. The official *ordonnance* of 29 December 1664 stated: 'the lords and gentlemen of the court and suite to whom His Majesty will have permitted by order or warrant signed by Himself and by one of the secretaries of state, the right to wear gold and silver in either

galloon, lace or embroidery upon the said coats.'

As the new coats had to be granted by special warrant they were known as *justaucorps à brevet*, warrant coats. Louis XIV did not actually sign any

34 Claude Hallé, 'The Doge of Genoa Making His Apologies to Louis XIV', 1685.

In order to detach the Republic of Genoa from her alliance with Spain Louis XIV sent his fleet to bombard the port into submission. On hearing that the Doge never officially left his city, Louis XIV ordered him to be brought to Versailles. Doge Imperiale Lercari was received in the Galerie des Glaces with all the silver plate and the silver throne on display, and had to crave forgiveness, on 16 May 1685. The Dogal robes were of red velvet and his senators wore black. (*Musée des Beaux Arts, Marseilles; cliché des Musées Nationaux*)

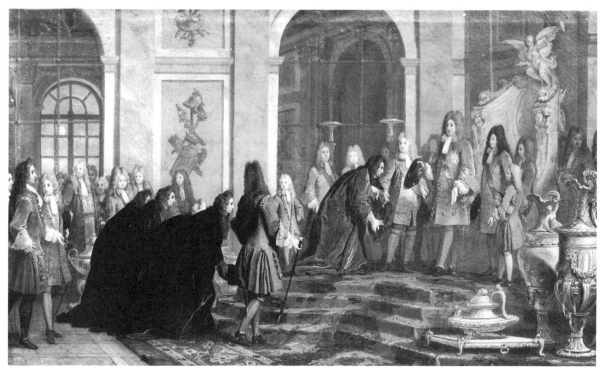

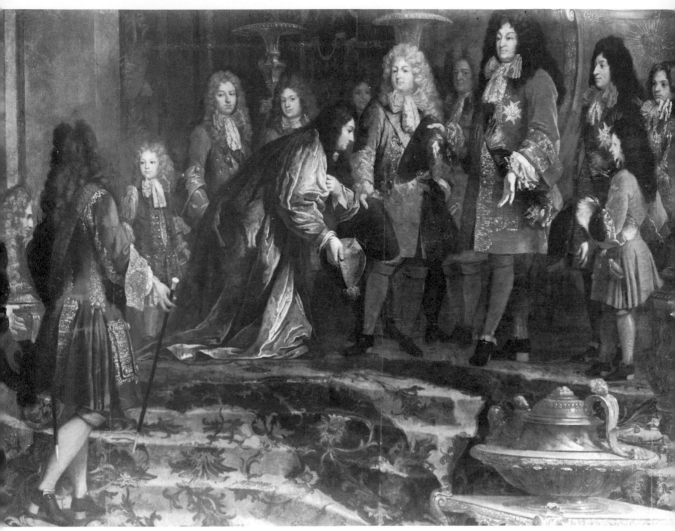

warrants until 4 February 1665, when they were
countersigned by the secretary of state, Guénégaud.[1]
This achieved the effect of creating a uniform which
princes and dukes would beg for the right to wear, and
continued throughout the reign. The provost the
Marquis de Sourches noted religiously in his journals
who had just died and who was receiving his right to
wear a *justaucorps à brevet*, as matters of some
consequence. The coat was blue lined with scarlet
and was worn with a waistcoat, both being
embroidered with gold and a little silver thread in a
particular pattern. It was restricted to the king, the
royal family and princes of the blood, and to the listed
members. Wearers could join royal excursions to
Saint Germain or Versailles without an invitation, and
the coat could be worn for second or third mourning,
but not for full first mourning. Saint Simon did not

35 Charles LeBrun, 'The Doge of Genoa Making His
Apologies to Louis XIV', 1685.

LeBrun's more detailed depiction shows the grand
chamberlain with the cane wearing the *justaucorps à brevet*,
which has the special embroidery up the seams, round the
sleeve head, and down the coat tails and pockets. This style
of embroidery affected courts all round Europe. The
picture supports Saint Simon's statement that he never saw
Louis XIV or his brother in the justaucorps, for none of the
royals are shown wearing it. Louis XIV has embroidery
down the front and on the cuff but not down the seams. This
also applies to his brother Philippe Duc d'Orléans to the
king's right, with his son the Duc de Chartres. On the king's
left is the Grand Dauphin with blond hair, and his son
Bourgogne. The 1680s introduced vertical pockets, and the
number of bows behind a cravat was increased to four or
five. Louis required himself to be portrayed taller than he
really was, for his son was actually taller than he. (*Versailles,
photograph Giraudon*)

appear at court until 1691 and said that he never saw Louis XIV or his brother Monsieur in the coat. The Dauphin once he had reached adulthood was allowed a justaucorps of his own in brown embroidered with silver, which he granted to his friends who rode with him to hunt wolves, but he also distributed the coat to non-hunting associates. On 1 February 1688 Louis XIV said he was tired of seeing so many brown coats of the Dauphin's pattern about the palace and told him to restrict the wearing strictly to his hunting companions, so Monseigneur the Dauphin had to devise a new one, still in brown. The blue coat remained the most coveted, and on 22 September 1691 Sourches recorded that the Maréchal de la Feuillade had just died and his coat right had been transferred to the Marquis de la Salle, a master of the royal wardrobe. It is significant that the justaucorps first appeared in 1665 when Louis XIV revived the Order of St Michael, restricted to 100 members who had to be Roman Catholics. They were both honours to bewitch the ambitious, and both put the wearer to some expense.[2] A national style for men also emerged, for Louis XIV was so attached to petticoat breeches during the first two decades of his adulthood that he was obliged to shorten his coats, otherwise he would have looked like a triangle with the bottom of the coat stuck out over the petticoat fullness. The British more sensibly had gone over to narrow kneebreeches under their coats, after the Spanish type, but Louis, it seems, was too fond of the swirl and sway of petticoats, so he shortened his coats to the hip. Such short coats were dubbed *l'habit à la française*, as they were regarded as particularly French.[3] It was mentioned in Chapter 1 that when Henriette Anne visited Dover the shortness of her courtiers' coats was criticized and mocked. On horseback the tails of the short French coat needed to be pulled aside which led to their being buttoned up, and it became a feature to show the lining, with, say, a scarlet lining lighting the rear of a gold coat. These *habits à la française* were adopted by the cavalry in the next century as they were less impeding than the full-skirted coats of the early 1700s, and were an early form of 'bum freezer'.

With the ladies Louis XIV faced a more complicated situation. As they were not admitted to knightly orders, and could not serve in areas where they might attain distinction as a general, admiral, governor or ambassador, it was not possible to devise an order or a *justaucorps* for them. It was all very well directing them to appear at court in the height of fashion, but there were a few who flatly refused to do

so. The king's own sister-in-law Madame, Elisabeth Charlotte, wore her scarlet hunting suit as much as possible, preferring the hip-length coat and full skirts to being corseted into a boned bodice and hung about with hip pads. The Princesse de Soubise, with whom Louis XIV had an *affaire*, refused to follow the fashion for hoisting up the skirt to show the petticoats as she was afraid of getting a chill in her kidneys. A health fanatic, she lived on a diet of salad, chicken and veal to avoid overheating the body which she felt might give her a red nose, although it did not prolong her span on earth. Saint Simon says that her signal to the king that her husband was going to be away for the night was to wear a pair of emerald earrings. Then there was that hoyden, the king's cousin La Grande Mademoiselle, Anne Marie Louise Duchesse de Montpensier, with her fondness for mock heroics and military dress. Faced with these individuals the king would have to be very careful about interfering with feminine attire, but he did become increasingly impatient with the developments of the 1670s. He did not object greatly to the slimmer line with all fullness now placed below the hips, but he did dislike the vogue for *manteaux* or mantos. These unboned garments were like nightgowns or Indian gowns in construction, they covered the shoulders and they were not sculpted into a rigid bodice, so that they had an air of undress about them which the king did not think right for a court. He wanted formality, grandeur, dignity when his ladies were on parade.

Fortunately for Louis XIV Madame Elisabeth Charlotte agreed with him. The memoirs of the period do not bother to state who was involved in the creation of the *grand habit* for women, but as Madame was such a strong advocate of this court dress, and her husband Monsieur Philippe was so keen on anything to do with clothes, some discussions between Louis XIV and the Orléans household were likely. Saint Simon says that Madame was very much a princess of the old school, fiercely attached to honour, virtue, rank and greatness, so she would have had firm opinions on the subject of a dignified costume for women. In addition Saint Simon informs us that after supper Louis XIV liked to lean against the balustrade in front of his state bed, to comment on the clothes and appearances of the princes and princesses who had supped with him, and now stood in half-circle to receive his approbation or criticism. This was another occasion when discussion about reforming women's dress at court could have taken place. It was not a subject for official publications. To date I have not

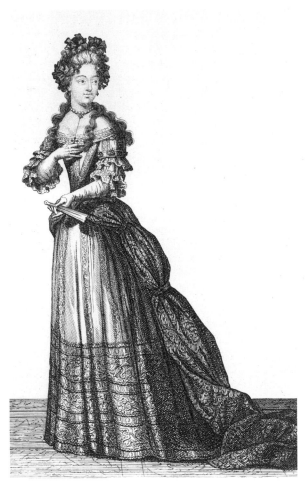

36 'Lady in the Grand Habit', *c.* 1682.
The *grand habit* for ladies retained the bare shoulders of the
1660s which mantos had concealed in the 1670s, and kept
the short cap sleeve of about 1672. It was a deliberate
attempt to freeze a fashion into a permanent official uniform
for women at court, and was imitated across Europe. The
boned bodice was never altered, but the skirt could follow
the modes. The bows in the hair reflect the style launched
by the Duchesse de Fontanges. (*Stadtmuseum, Munich*)

found an order in the *Gazette de France* banning
mantos from court. They were at the height of fashion
and became established as the dominant garment for
women for the remainder of the reign. To the surprise
of Louis XIV the fact that he did not like them made
no impact beyond the court; the town adored them.
They represented a more casual look after the fiercely
boned bodices of the 1660s and '70s. A small corset
was necessary underneath but that was all, and a
stomacher had to be developed to conceal the front of
the corset, for there was a gap occasioned by the wrap-
over nature of the dressing-gown-like manto, which
was fastened by a sash. A distinction began to arise
between *habit de ville*, town dress, the mode, and
unfashionable, conservative *grand habit*, court dress.
What the king wanted was for women to continue to
wear the bare-shouldered, boned bodices of his
youth, so the *grand habit* retained the features of the
1670s from which it emerged. It had short cap sleeves
which were the dominant type of woman's sleeve in
the decade, a long, boned bodice, and a small lace
fichu around the shoulder. The skirt could follow the
fashionable line, so that it was pulled back to show the
petticoat. As the cap sleeve was short the sleeve of the
shift had to be dressed up for court appearances, so it
was given two layers of frills, termed the *engageantes*,
pointing in opposite directions. Madame wore the
grand habit all the time she was not in hunting livery.
It was the uniform she craved, which saved her the
time and trouble of having to decide what to wear
every day for the evening entertainments. She was
most indignant in 1694 when a report from Berlin
claimed that she wore mantos. She wrote back to
Germany immediately that she had never worn a
manto in her life! She said people looked like
chambermaids in mantos, she found them
uncomfortable and complicated with the stomacher,
corset and manto; too many layers, she said. Madame
endorsed the *grand habit* with enthusiasm. The
earliest visual example is datable to about 1683, by
which time Madame was in her thirties, a respectable
wife and mother, so she wore her *grand habits* in black
cloth, with only the petticoat in gold or silver; this set
the style for older women. The younger generation
could wear the whole garment in cloth of gold or
silver. The bare shoulders pleased the king, and
provided a good background for pearls and diamonds,
but bare shoulders were a distinct disadvantage in
winter. On a very cold 3 February 1695, Louis XIV
told off Madame for wearing a scarf with her *grand
habit* at high mass in the Chapel Royal, but she
retorted that she preferred to be badly dressed than to
freeze. The shoulders of the other ladies were turning
blue with cold.[4] This typified Louis XIV's
inconsiderate attitude towards women, which
incensed Saint Simon:

Whether pregnant, ill, less than six weeks after a delivery,
and whatever the ferocity of the weather, they had to be in
the *grand habit*, dressed and laced into their corsets, to go to
Flanders, or farther still, to dance, to stay up, attend
festivities, eat, be gay and good company, change locations,
without appearing afraid, nor incommoded by heat, cold,

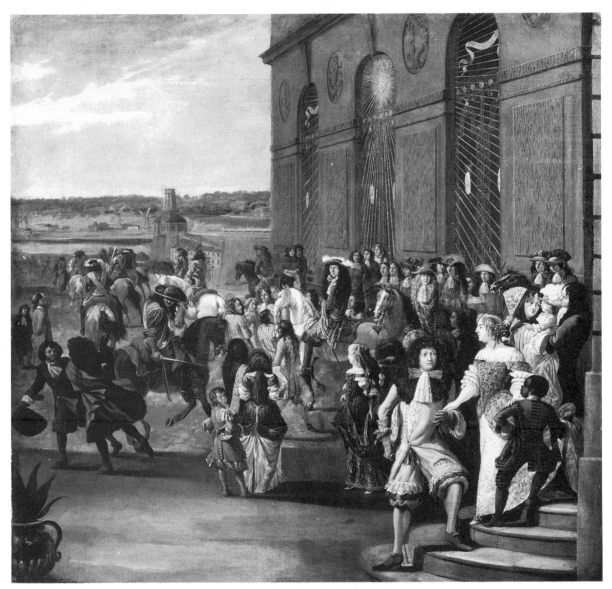

air, dust, and all that precisely on the days and the times directed without disturbing arrangements for so much as a minute.

Louis loved to travel from seat to seat in a coach crowded with women but now they all had to be in court dress, and the unfortunate queen could find herself squeezed between mistresses, bastards and nurses. The discomfort of court life was illustrated by the Duchesse de Chevreuse who on one such journey from Versailles to Fontainebleau was taken by a need to relieve herself, but the king did not think about women's shorter plumbing, and did not stop the coach once. The duchesse had to writhe all the way to the

37 French School, 'Louis XIV visiting the Grotto of Thetis', *c.* 1683.
The lady on the steps shows the *grand habit* as it became fixed, with four tiers of frills on the shift sleeve, the top tier the opposite way round to the others. As the lady's train requires a page to hold it up, it looks long enough for her to be a duchess. Black pageboys were fashionable after a North African king sent one named Osmin as a present. The grooms in front of Louis XIV's white horse all have braided liveries. Having built the Grotto the king later knocked it down as Versailles expanded. (*Versailles, cliché des Musées Nationaux*)

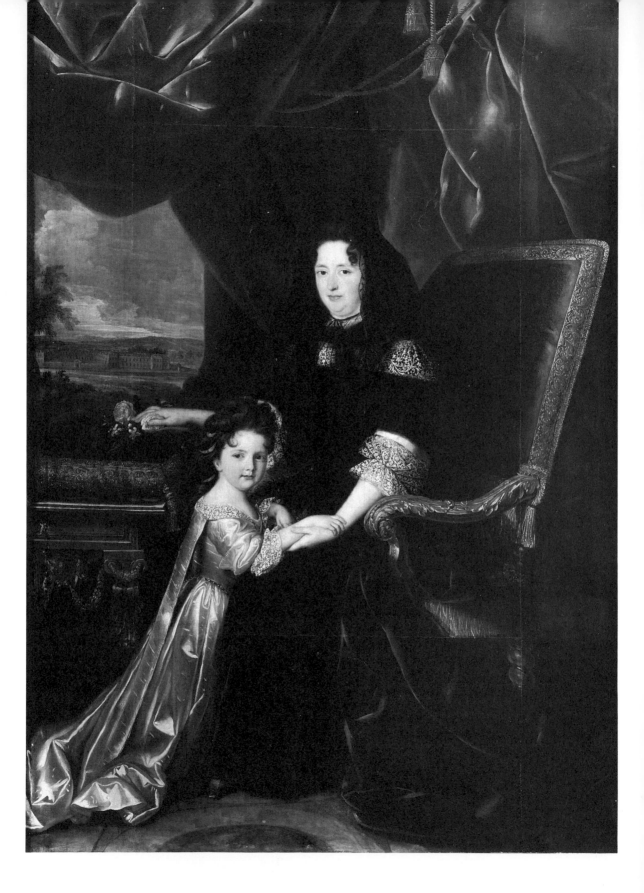

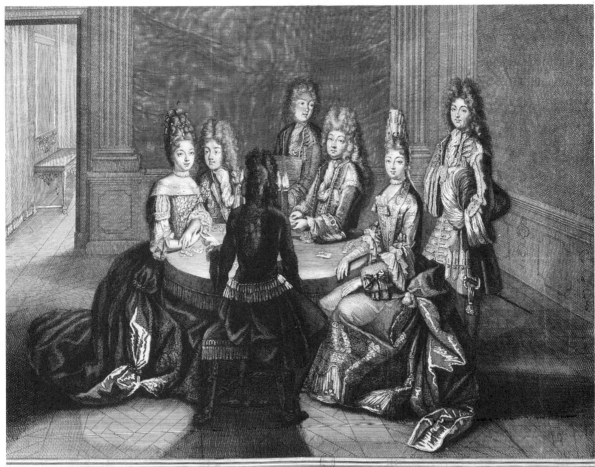

SECONDE CHAMBRE DES APARTEMENS.

Monseigneur.
Madame la Princesse de Conty Douairiere .

Grané par Fais par A. Trouvain avec & Augois au grand Masque par almand les Mathurins Auec privilège du Roy.

3. Monsieur le Duc de Bourbon .
4. Madame la Duchesse de Bourbon.
5. Monsieur de Vandôme, grand Prieur de France .

OPPOSITE
38 Ferdinand Elle, 'Marquise de Maintenon with her Niece'.
Louis XIV's morganatic second wife wore the *grand habit* in black or brown. She considered bare shoulders immodest, so she carried the lace fichu up to her throat. She had a sobering influence upon the king's appearance and lifestyle. (*Versailles, cliché des Musées Nationaux*)

39 André Trouvain, 'Seconde Chambre des Apartemens', 1696.
The distinction between the *grand habit* and *habit de ville*. Court dress as worn by the Duchesse de Bourbon, on the left, has bare shoulders above a lace fichu, a boned bodice and cap sleeves, and the hair is dressed into a firmament. The Dowager Princesse de Conti on the right wears the fashionable manto with long sleeves which cover the shoulders, and a commode headdress, plus elegant gloves, a muff and face patches. The Dauphin has a towering periwig which cannot quite match the height of the commodes. An *apartemens* was an evening reception. (*Bibliothèque Nationale, Paris*)

oval court at Fontainebleau, when she asked the Duc de Beauvillier to stand guard, as she dashed into the nearest edifice, the chapel, to burst.[5]

At first there was some confusion about where the *grand habit* had to be worn. Madame wrote that it was compulsory at Versailles as the royal residence, but not at other châteaux like Fontainebleau and Marly le Roi, yet Saint Simon mentions one occasion at Fontainebleau when the king got angry because the women were wearing mantos. They had not changed into the *grand habit* to watch the evening comedy with the king but were sidling off in evident hope of missing the duty. Four words from Louis brought them back, and they changed into formal dress. But by now even he had felt some need for relaxation from the clockwork routine of Versailles, so he began to develop Marly in 1679. True to form he selected another boggy site, for the very name, from Meerlieu or Merelea, means a place with water. An informal

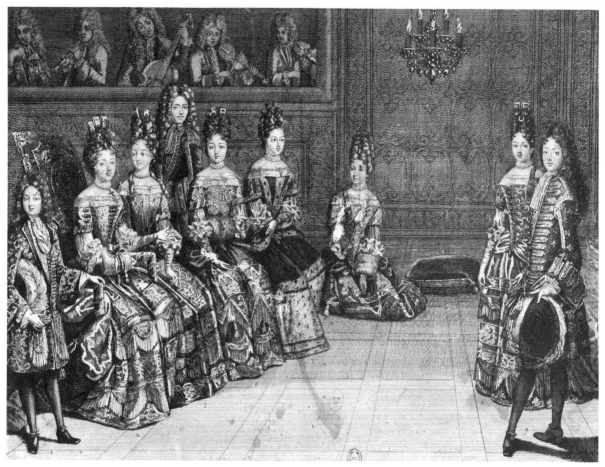

regime was established here, so ladies could wear mantos and not the *grand habit*. This was one reason why Madame declined to attend at first, and she also did not approve of the relaxation in etiquette which allowed people to be seated in the presence.

The *grand habit* made an enormous impact upon European courts right across to Russia. It was adopted by the majority, for it set a special standard of correct dress by which courts would be judged. The Spanish court style of farthingales for women received a serious blow, for even the Hapsburgs in Vienna were to adopt the *grand habit*. In France this court dress endured down to the Revolution, with the bodice fixed at a regulation pattern, although the skirts altered as the line grew wider into paniers. In the British court the *grand habit* was termed the *corps de robe* or stiff-bodied gown. The Spanish court tried to resist but in 1700 it was to get a French king, when the Spanish court dress was brought to an end and the *grand habit* was instituted for women. The French court did not allow any coverings on the head with the

40 André Trouvain, 'Quatrième Chambre des Apartemens', 1696.

The *grand habit* was compulsory wear in the state rooms at Versailles. The princess in the armchair is Madame, Elisabeth Charlotte Duchesse d'Orléans who adored the *grand habit*. Her son Philippe Duc de Chartres and his sister Elisabeth Charlotte (who became Duchess of Lorraine in 1698) are on the right. On Madame's left is her daughter-in-law, Louis XIV's bastard by Montespan, Françoise Marie de Bourbon, now Duchesse de Chartres; her face is covered with patches, whereas Madame and her children wear none. All the ladies have their hair up in firmaments, backed with ribbons, and fringes decorate most of the petticoats. The boy beside Madame is Louis Duc de Bourgogne, the king's eldest grandson. (*Bibliothèque Nationale, Paris*)

grand habit. Ribbons and jewels were permitted, but the late 1670s' vogue for lace pinners and caps was not allowed, so these formed the separate *habit de ville*. Thus the hair had to be displayed with the *grand habit*, regardless of what fashion was up to.

For those men not honoured by the *justaucorps à*

brevet court dress was simply a suit of quality in velvet or better. Madame de Montespan says that as Louis XIV approached his forties he began to simplify his flamboyant attire. The flowing plumes on his hat, the elaborate baldrics and riding boots embroidered with gold or silver, were all discarded.[6] 1678 was the year in which *Le Nouveau Mercure Galant* was allowed to illustrate the English suit as the ideal for men, and Louis XIV himself adopted the knee-length coat and waistcoat and the narrow kneebreeches. The outfit had now been around for 12 years so Louis had grown more accustomed to it, and perhaps he felt that its simplicity accorded better with his dignity as he entered middle age. Consequently, the English suit became correct dress for men at court, although the French were pretending it was theirs.

The Spanish government was having problems in ensuring that its colonies kept to Spanish dress for dignitaries. Madame d'Aulnoy reported: 'All the *Spanish* Officers at *Naples* were enjoyn'd to re-assume the *Spanish* Dress: 'Twas believed that the Neapolitans would soon imitate them; but seeing they did not in the least, an Ordinance was published, by the Sound of Trumpet, at the beginning of *August*, commanding all the Officers of Justice to Apparel themselves after the *Spanish* Fashion.' From Madrid she related 'We were here informed, that the Spanish Captains, who were at *Naples*, were not a little mortified at the Prohibition that was issued out to forbid them to go drest after the *French* fashion. There is never a *Spaniard* of 'em all that is not ravished with Joy, as soon as he is out of his own Country, to quit the Habit of it also.' This was in 1680, so the rot had started before the French takeover of the Spanish kingdom. Of course Madame d'Aulnoy was forced to don Spanish court dress in order to visit Queen Marie Louise. She knew it did not become her and thought the new queen was the only foreigner whom the Spanish style did suit.

The daughter of Monsieur and Henriette Anne was dressed in a Spanish gown of rose colour embroidered with silver, and had the simple Spanish hairstyle parted in the centre, with only one lock roped with pearls to her waist. The pendants in her ears, which reached to the breast, looked very heavy.[7] The new French queen of Spain was trying to look Spanish but her husband Carlos II was not so devoted to Spanish court dress. It had been instituted by Philip IV on 11 February 1623 and published in 1624 as the *Capitulos de Reformacion*, when he had banned sinful ruffs and ordered a plain collar of cardboard covered with linen; it had looked a conservative suit even then. The black doublet and black kneebreeches worn with the new golilla collar were looking antique by 1680. Coats were now the necessary dress for gentlemen, so many younger Spaniards felt that the court suit was too peculiar. Carlos II in particular disliked the hard collar, and from the age of nine had expressed a preference for the military cravat.[8]

The cravat was an English invention which arose during the Civil War. The royalists found their very wide lace collars a nuisance during battle so at first they tried to tame them by tying them together in front with a ribbon formed into a bow. Numerous examples were portrayed by the court painter William Dobson when Charles I transferred his capital to Oxford in 1642. Lord Byron, Sir Thomas Chicheley and Colonel John Russell were all painted with the bow of ribbon catching their lace collars in front. On the Continent the military preferred very small collars, but some of the English went even further and discarded collars altogether. Colonel Richard Neville favoured a collarless shirt and a scarf round his neck, held by a black bow, while an unknown officer, in a painting in the Tate Gallery, simply knotted the scarf itself in front, and discarded the ribbon bow. The cravat was born. It was strictly a military style in the 1640s. During the 1650s wide collars made a comeback but some officers kept to cravats. It was the French troops Louis XIV sent to help Portugal to defeat Spain in 1665 who introduced the military cravat to the Spanish peninsula. A Spanish regiment was formed on the French army model, with cravats, and young Carlos II loved cravats. The Spanish Regent the queen mother put her foot down and forced him into black suits and golillas, but once Carlos II was king and of age the occasions when he donned Spanish court dress diminished, although officials had to wear it. Clearly its days were numbered.[9] The influence of English suits and cravats adopted and promoted by the French court was too strong.

The vogue for masquerades and carrousels, or horse ballets, predated Louis XIV. His grandfather had started the Place Royale, now the Place des Vosges, in Paris as a parade ground for festivities. The first carrousel given there had been to celebrate the double marriages of Louis XIII, Anna Maria Mauritia, Elizabeth of France and Philip IV. As a boy Louis XIV had appeared as the sun god and other mythological deities in the court ballets given by his mother the

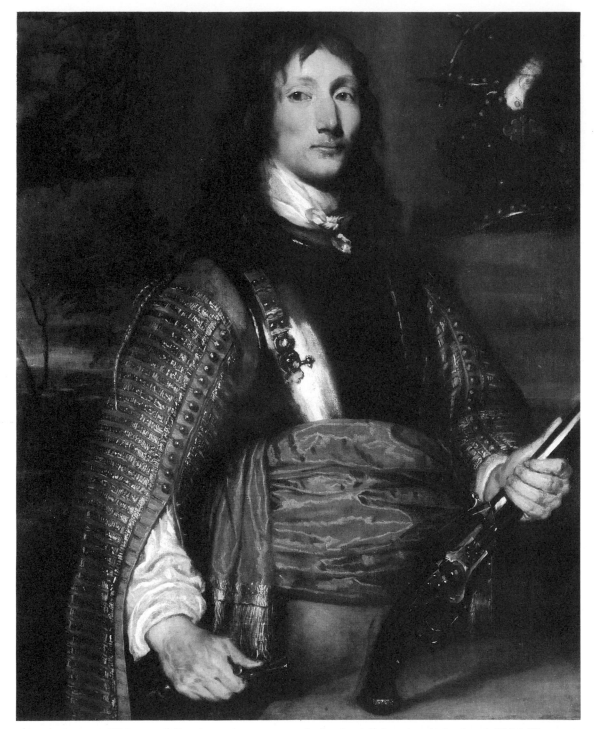

41 William Dobson, 'Unknown Officer'.

The established golilla collar at the Spanish court faced serious undermining by the informal cravat. This was an English invention that came about during the Civil War (1641/2–8) when Cavalier collars proved a nuisance and had to be tied down or else replaced. This officer sports a length of linen knotted in front as the first cravat. English exiles took the cravat to the Continent, where French regiments adopted it and conveyed it to Spain. Carlos II preferred cravats to golilla collars. (*Tate Gallery, London*)

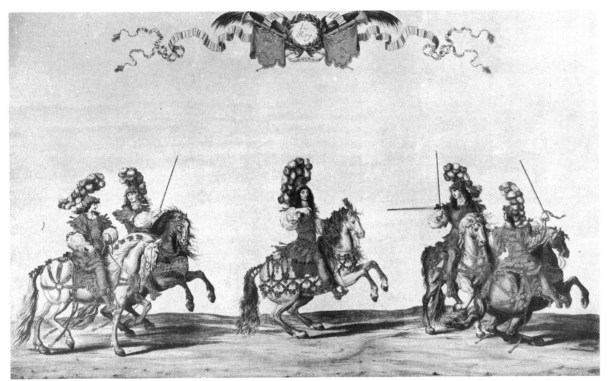

Regent, so this encouraged an interest in dressing up. In 1652 the young king asked the explorer François de la Boullaye le Gaitz to visit him in the Persian costume he had just brought back from a visit to Isfahan. He encouraged the publication of Ballaye's *Voyages et Observations* in 1653 with a plate of Persian dress, and in 1657 sent him back to Persia as French envoy with gifts for the Shah.[10] The English court was already familiar with Persian dress for Van Dyck had painted both Sir Robert Shirley, the Englishman who represented Persia in Europe, and his Persian wife Teresia in 1622, as well as the Earl of Denbigh, master of the great wardrobe, in 1633 wearing the Indian pyjamas he had purchased on his visit to that country. The East India Company and the Dutch equivalent were both importing exotic goods before Louis XIV was born, so he was participating in an established fashion for exotica.

A mammoth carrousel was staged in 1662 to celebrate the birth of the Dauphin in 1661. Louis XIV was the Emperor of the Romans, for he saw himself as an imperial idol, and Monsieur Philippe was the King of the Persians, although the costume was much shorter than those worn in Persia. The Duc de Guise was King of the Americas, a title the English and Spanish would have disputed, but his costume was pure Roman armour, with a quantity of ostrich plumes

42 Jacques Bailly, 'Louis XIV as the Roman Emperor in the Grand Carrousel of 1662', gouache upon engravings by I. Silvestre, F. Chauveau and J. Le Pautre, published 1670. The elaborate horse ballet was mounted to celebrate the birth of the Dauphin. Louis XIV's Roman armour was covered with diamonds, and he claimed to be more famous than ancient Romans. The celebrations included tournaments as well, mixing medieval tradition with classical. (*Versailles*)

cascading from his helmet as the slightest indication of an American Indian chief's eagle-feathered war bonnet. His followers wore animal skins and bare arms to indicate savagery, but the trumpeters' costumes and shell-like helmets seemed more oceanic than native. A strong Roman look flavoured representations of American Indians in the Baroque period because the Roman period had been the only one Europeans knew about which had used semi-naked clothes, so they were only able to design American naked tribes in a Roman manner. It sufficed to give them a lot of feathers. That was well understood to be Indian, but in Europe it had to be ostrich plumes as these were the most expensive and superior type of feathers.

The king's outfit was described by Father Menestrier in his treatise on jousts, tourneys and carrousels of 1669. The Roman armour had three

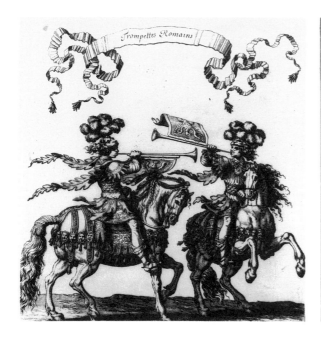

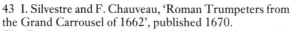

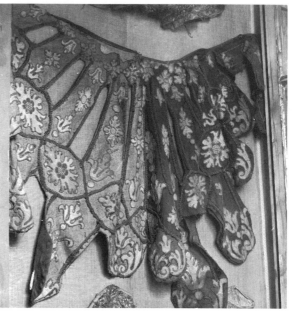

43 I. Silvestre and F. Chauveau, 'Roman Trumpeters from the Grand Carrousel of 1662', published 1670.
The Roman armour is decked with flying pendants in the dagged late Gothic taste, which can also be seen in the waist pendants. This shows how the medieval concept of the herald still influenced the designer of the whole production, Henri Gissey. (*Versailles*)

44 Waist Pendants.
These surviving waist pendants in two-tone medieval pattern *mi parti*, show what the pendants in the Grand Carrousel were like, but whether these are the ones which were worn there is uncertain. They were conserved at the Ecole Militaire at Beaumont-en-Ange, so they may have been handed down to the Army to use on gala days. (*Musée du Vieux Honfleur, Honfleur, Calvados*)

bands of roses of diamonds, 26 extraordinarily large diamonds and three large diamond clasps. There were 44 diamond roses on the gorget, and a dozen on the strip sleeves, the *lambrequins*, and ten chains each with a pendant with diamonds and other stones. Forty scales garnished with diamonds were attached to the strips. Fifty-two chains ornamented the upper sleeve and the sash, and 24 diamonds towered up both sides of the sleeves. His breeches were covered by 40 lambrequins, composed of chains of diamonds, each ending in a pendant. The headdress was a golden helmet decorated with more diamonds, with a prodigious centrepiece decked with two great diamonds, and a dozen pink diamonds, and topped with a magnificent bouquet of ostrich plumes in flame tone, with a black aigrette.

Monsieur's Persian vest was scarlet covered with rubies and diamonds upon silver embroidery. Down the front and sleeves were many buttonholes outlined with the same gems, and the top and bottom of the sleeves were decorated with chains, rubies and diamonds. The outfit was further enlivened by an infinity of knots in scarlet and white ribbon. On his

head was a Persian crown decked with rubies and diamonds, and topped by a great number of scarlet and white plumes with aigrettes of which one was composed entirely of rubies and diamonds. The sabre had a mixture of gems up the scabard, and chains, diamonds and rubies bedecked the handle. The boots had emblems on the front and were smothered with gems of prodigious size.

There was a Turkish entry led by Monsieur le Prince in a turban covered with precious stones, and garnished with white, black and blue plumes, with a great aigrette attached by a brooch of diamonds. His followers wore trousers and caftans. The whole costume extravaganza was designed by Henri Gissey. Menestrier stressed that variety of costume was essential for a good carrousel, which contained quadrilles performed by groups of horsemen. Pages should be in trunkhose, trumpeters in cassocks with hanging sleeves, heralds in tunics with the coats of arms of the provinces on the front and back. There should be an element of contest between opposing sides who should both be in fanciful armour based on the Roman model, with a cuirass over a leather tunic, whose sleeves and hem were cut into strips, under which a skirt should be worn. The heroes' helmets should be embroidered fabric surmounted by quantities of ostrich plumes, although Turks and Moors should have turbans, Russians and Poles fur hats. Richness should be aimed for. He remembered favourably the royal cavalcade of 1656 when 16 pages in masks had liveries of cloth of gold and silver upon a ground of pink and white. Their hats were in cloth of silver with waving plumes, and their stockings were silk. The boots were of gauze with white shoes decked with pink. They rode expensive horses, with saddles of gold and silver decoration, and the horses' tails were tied with a great number of ribbons in pink and white. On this occasion Louis XIV had also appeared as a Roman hero with a helmet of golden gauze decked with diamonds. Louis XIV participated in many such carrousels in the 1650s and 1660s, but by the 1680s when he had begun to have the gout, he directed others to stage them and became a spectator. There were plenty of books to consult for exotic subjects. Vincent Le Blanc's *World Surveyed*, translated into English in 1660, described the clothes of Bengal, Arabia, Ethiopia and Mexico.

---

45 Imitation Roman armour.
The Roman outfits were decorated with the same richness which characterized Baroque embroidery on clothes. For the royals the decoration was in gold and silver with jewels. This humbler version is decked with copper wire and copper sequins to shine more cheaply. It gives a good indication of the weight of clothes about which Madame kept complaining at court. (*Musée du Vieux Honfleur*)

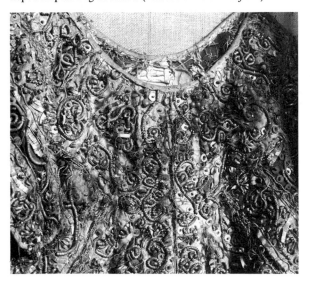

In London Charles II's cosmographer John Ogilby published his illustrated tomes on *China* 1669, *Africa* 1670, *America* 1671, and *Asia* 1673, so designers like Gissey and Berain did not lack for source material.[11]

The period saw a strange amalgam, which reached as far as Ireland, of medieval chivalry and imperial Roman grandeur, with the aristocracy staging jousts and tournaments while dressed as Roman generals and emperors. Some noble houses still retained their fools. Charles II had his fool in Thomas Killigrew whose livery allowance for two years at a time was 30 yards of velvet, 16 yards of damask and 36 yards of fringe, in 1661.[12] Thus there was an overlap of medieval traditions with the Roman ideals of the Baroque. In the 1640s the Comte de Gramont and his friend Matta sported green and blue as the favoured colours of their ladies. On her visit to the English court of Charles II the Comtesse d'Aulnoy encountered two champions of chivalry in the elderly Duke and Duchess of Newcastle. The king was entertaining the Prince of Neuburg, and decided to take him to a ball at Hampton Court. The royal barges set off along the Thames, which the comtesse considered the handsomest river in the world, accompanied by musicians playing a symphony upon trumpets, drums, flutes, violins, theorbos and cymbals, with voices. The barges were covered with Persian carpets, and hung with brocaded tapestries in rose. Suddenly they were intercepted by two barges. The first contained 'antick knights' with a hero in the centre in full armour, and a pavilion of green and gold in which was the portrait of a lady. The second barge was occupied by Diana and her hunting nymphs who all held arrows and had quivers on their backs. The goddess was attired in rich clothes and jewels, but the comtesse commented 'that there never was so aged a *Diana* seen before; however, she had certain ruins of Beauty which were more valuable than all her Attire.' The Prince of Neuburg thought they must be actors but the hero was rowed across and proved to be the Duke of Newcastle who produced a small picture of his duchess and challenged the court to deny her beauty. Charles II replied that no lady present could possibly excel the duchess in looks, so the duke allowed the barges to proceed. The Newcastles went as far as acting out tales of romance with the duchess as a princess of the Enchanted Palace or the invisible Isle who had to be rescued by the Knight of the Wood, namely her husband. They employed actors to assist them in these fantasies, and were possibly the last exponents of medieval chivalry on the grand scale to perform in the woods of their estates without an audience. The carrousels of Louis XIV were mounted in public.[13]

During her short life Monsieur's first wife Henriette Anne was the centre of chivalrous gestures at the French court. The minister Hugues de Lionne estimated that entertaining the court was going to cost him 25–30,000 livres in 1659, for it involved balls, ballets, comedies, games, fireworks and an open table. When they were young Louis XIV and Henrietta Anne loved dressing up, and twice at Fontainebleau in 1661 the Lionnes were surprised in bed by masked invaders who proved to be the king and his sister-in-law enjoying some high jinks. Money rolled, wrote the Abbé de Choisy. Purses were open, the king wanted joy and abundance, and lawyers could always find money for young aristocrats. The rates of interest were hard, but what did the young care about conditions?[14] The magnificent but fatal fête at Vaux-le-Vicomte presented by Fouquet was in honour of the first Madame Henriette Anne who arrived in a litter. She was more charming than the Spanish queen, for Henriette Anne had grown up in France, spoke the language and knew the society, whereas Marie Thérèse still had not mastered French, loathed French cooking, and in many ways remained a childlike character, a convent innocent, where her sister-in-law had known exile and the execution of her father Charles I. Henriette Anne was Diana in the *Ballet des Saisons* at Fontainbleau on 23 July 1661, and she was chief shepherdess in the *Ballet des Arts* at the Louvre on 8 January 1663, when she wore a straw hat covered with flowers. She also appeared as Pallas Athene in classical dress and wearing a helmet, with four Amazon maidens as her suite. In 1666 she was a shepherdess again in the *Ballet des Muses* when she appeared with her pet spaniel Mimi, and wore a pale green shift edged with emeralds and pearls. Her health, however, was always fragile, and she soon tired, so her participation had to be limited. Her successor the second Madame, Elisabeth Charlotte, did not participate in ballets; she preferred her hounds and horses, and loathed having to attend the king's masquerade parties.[15]

In September 1670 Charles II sent the second Duke of Buckingham to thank Louis XIV for his condolences over the death of his sister Henriette Anne, which the duke had considered worth going to war over. During dinner a masked cavalier and two masked ladies started to dance, and were then joined

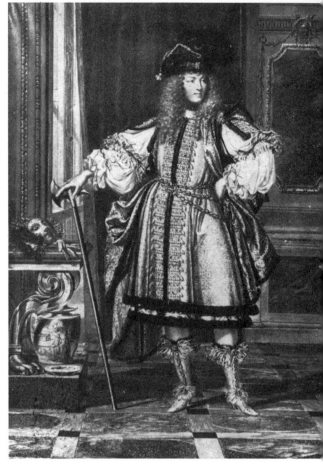

46 Henri Gissey, 'Louis XIV as a Hungarian'.
This is a masquerade costume; the mask is on the table. The braided fastening is Hungarian but the sleeves are in the fashion of about 1666. There is a cloak of sorts with two hems matching the two hems on the coat, but its draped effect is not Hungarian. A masquerade costume usually only takes a few details from an original. (*Gallice Sale, 25 May 1934*)

by other ladies. The cavalier wore a glittering sword and baldric which the *Gazette* valued at 20,000 écus. The ladies all admired the sword and tried to take it off the cavalier; they succeeded and presented it to Buckingham. The cavalier said it was a gift, and proved to be Louis XIV once he removed his mask. This elaboration of a simple presentation typified the king's taste and policy. Any activity at his court had to be surrounded with complicated courtesy and orchestrated into a ceremony.

Staged masques had become too expensive, and masquerade balls were much cheaper for the Crown because all the guests paid for their own costumes, balls did not last too long. When Elisabeth Charlotte arrived in 1671 balls still lasted until dawn. The changing of clothes during the ball was quite common. Lady Mary Bertie observed of a grand ballet at the English court in February 1670–1 that the guests 'shifted their clothes three times'. The international character was always strong. In February 1667 the *Gazette de France* reported that Louis XIV had worn a costume that was half Persian and half Chinese, but that the Duc de Saint Aignan was completely Persian. In London Peregrine Bertie

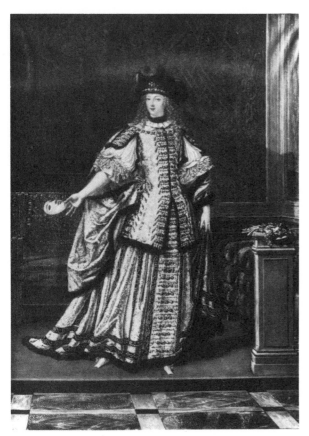

47 'Louise de la Vallière as a Hungarian'.
Gissey clearly designed the costumes as a pair, presenting the king and his mistress as a Hungarian couple with matching fur trim and braid. Her cloak, like his, is more designed than East European. (*Gallice Sale, 25 May 1934*)

48 Pierre Mignard, 'Henriette Anne Duchesse d'Orléans'. The English princess starred in many French court productions and masquerades. This costume takes the peasant woman's jacket and skirt and elaborates them into a pseudo-Roman bodice with the basques stiffened out like Roman *pteruges*, while the skirt is panelled with jewels. It may be the outfit the Duchesse wore in the *Ballet des Muses* of 1666 when she appeared with her miniature spaniel Mimi, for the green shift of a shepherdess can just be seen at the neckline. (*Duke of Northumberland*)

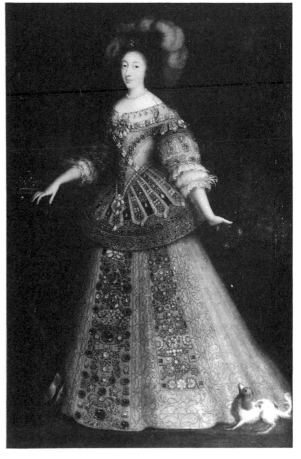

whereas a production came out of the budget of the great wardrobe. The term masquerade emerged about 1587, and masquerade balls were in existence by 1597. Fifty years later they had begun to replace masques, and were popular across Europe. *Les Nouvelles Ordinaires* of 18 June 1668 reported the masked ball given by the Queen Regent of Sweden where the king dressed as a Pole, the queen as a Turk, and the rest of the court as other nations. The Dauphin adored masked balls, and Madame de la Fayette recorded in 1688–9 'It is Monseigneur's pleasure at a ball to change his clothes frequently for the more joy of being unrecognised, and of talking to unimportant people. The court balls were so melancholy that they did not begin till almost midnight, and they were always over before two o'clock.'[16] By the time the Dauphin was a young man Louis XIV was showing signs of middle age so the wrote to the Countess of Rutland on 2 February 1685–6:

'The grate ball or masque att Court. . . There was to be in all twelve couples, each woman after a severall country fashion, and the men to have the habits of the same country as their partners, the Duke of Northumberland and my Lady Grafton Spaniards, my Lord Manchester and my Lady Derby Grecians, my Lord Dumblain and Miss Fox Moores, my Lord Litchfield and my Lady Walgrave Shepherds. I have not yet heard the other habits but they were all given them by the Queen.'[17]

The country of the shepherds was doubtless Arcadia. This seems to have been a group of masquerade dancers appearing at an ordinary ball, where the rest of the guests were not in costume, to perform an interlude organized by the queen. It usually fell to the queen to arrange the costuming: the Comte de Gramont had found in 1664–5 that Catherine of Braganza decided who should wear what for her masquerade. He would have liked to have attended as a Roman, but found that Lord Thanet was going to be Julius Caesar, and Prince Rupert of the Rhine (Elisabeth Charlotte's uncle) wanted to be Alexander, so it could be an area of dispute. Gramont notes a cruel joke played on Lady Muskerry, who was sent a fake note from the queen instructing her to come as a Babylonian. Her ladyship did not find it easy to obey: 'If you knew what a plague it is to find out, in this cursed town, in what manner the people of Babylon dress, you would pity me.' The comte said her solution was a sight to behold – 60 ells of gauze and silver tissue, with a sort of pyramid on her head adorned with a hundred thousand baubles.[18] That was not too far out, for Turkish sultanas wore a high headdress, so Lady Muskerry approached the correct outline. There was an international craze for masquerades with people dressed as east Europeans, Spaniards, Turks, Moors, Persians, Indians and Chinese, as well as characters from the *commedia dell'arte* and opera. The less dressed nations like black Africa and the Amazon Indians were not considered suitable, as their minimal costumes exposed too much flesh. The whole point of the exercise was to show off rich fabrics, bejewelled costumes, and the elaboration of what might in the country of origin have been quite a simple garment. It was another way to ensure that courtiers spent their money. The variety could be so great that in London Peregrine Bertie excused himself from sending the Countess of Rutland a complete account: 'I am very sorry that I cannot oblige your Ladyship with a relation of the severale dresses

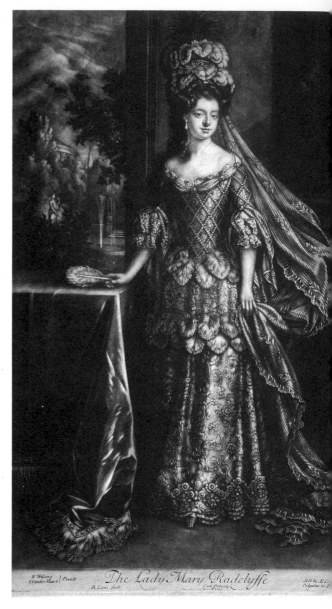

49 B. Lens after Wissing and Vander Vart, 'Lady Mary Radclyffe', *c.* 1695.

Masquerades were the subject of reports in the new newspapers, and *Le Nouveau Mercure Galant* reported them monthly. Courtiers exchanged letters describing costumes and preparations, and visited foreign courts to gather reports on the festivities. There was stiff competition between the English, Scandinavian and German courts to equal the glories of Versailles. Thus Lady Mary has ropes of pearls about her bodice, ostrich plumes at her head, waist and hip, and sumptuous petticoat with an appliquéd hem, to equal the French. (*National Portrait Gallery*) att my Lord Devonshire's ball, the variety was so greate that it prevented my remembering any particular habit.'

A number of masquerading costumes have survived in the royal collection in Denmark at Castle Rosenborg, from the reign of Christian V (1646–99). A jousting coat of 1685 in white satin heavily embroidered with gold intended for the king's birthday joust survived because the joust was cancelled when the queen died. The impact of French engravings can be seen in a white satin doublet embroidered with gold which was based upon the plate of Berain's design for Endymion in Lully's *Le Triomphe d'Amour* of 1681, although it lacks the pleated skirt of the original. A Polish coat in crimson velvet was worn by Christian V at a masquerade on 23 November 1687. A jousting coat of red cloth from about the same date is embroidered with a scroll pattern and gold relief embroidery, and lined with white satin patterned with red stems and gold sunflowers. There is also a costume worn by Frederick IV in 1710 as a Venetian valet, consisting of a doublet, waistcoat and kneebreeches, but not in a valet's textiles, for it is cloth of silver edged with a reddish-brown velvet and trimmed with a gold band. The cap is in the same velvet. There is also a collection of nightgowns (dressing gowns) where a damask coat is described as *japonisk*; this refers to the Japanese coats which the Dutch imported from the Far East, although the English called them Indian gowns. Other examples, however, which are of this oriental type were usually called Polish in Denmark, suggesting the land route as the principal source.[19]

Nothing survives of Louis XIV's magnificence, but the Ecole Militaire at Beaumont-en-Auge conserved some pieces of costume from carrousels, while Berain's patterns or choreography for the horse quadrilles survive in the National Museum in Stockholm. The waist pendants in particular resemble closely those worn by the Roman trumpeters, in the great carrousel of 1662, while the doublets smothered in wire, sequins, coils and whirls give an idea of the elaborate splendour of the original productions, although they lack the diamonds and pearls worn by the leading royals. They are now in the Musée du Vieux Honfleur. For lesser characters copper was used instead of gold, and rock crystal instead of diamonds, so that they would reflect something of the brilliance of the King Sun himself, although sumptuary law did not allow them the actual splendour worn by the monarch. The intention to dazzle was carried out to the full, with cloth of gold and silver with real diamonds for the leading royal participants, and copper and crystal for the rest, together with a huge quantity of ostrich plumes.

A masquerade party for the Dauphin was given on the last Sunday of the carnival season in February 1679. The Chevalier Colbert dressed as a Moorish slave and carried the train of the Duchess de Fontages, but *Le Nouveau Mercure Galant*'s report was so busy describing who was there, and who led whom in, that all it could say about the costumes was that they were 'designs of a magnificence and invention quite extraordinary'. The Dauphin danced until 2 a.m. and then changed back into French fashion. The journal, however, devoted much more room to describing the king's masquerade, because it had to. Louis XIV gave a series of balls that season in the Salle des Balets at the Château of Saint Germain. The Monday ball was masked. Louis XIV wore a vest of cloth of gold, and a cape of gold and silver Spanish point lace, a hat covered with flame plumes, and a black aigrette that had cost over 400 louis of gold. He did not wear a mask himself but the flame plumes would have betrayed his identity anyway. Queen Marie Thérèse came as a Persian, with a veiled face and the greater part of the crown jewels embroidered all over her costume. The Dauphin Louis was a North African or Moor with a flame-coloured corselet from which fell a black velvet drapery lined with flame, and embroidered with little golden flowers and diamonds. His hanging sleeves were of gold. He wore two skirts in the Roman manner, the top one in blue – embroidered with gold, and held open by diamond buttons. A cloak of French point lace in gold and silver was attached by clasps to his left shoulder and right hip. A small turban topped with plumes of flame and white graced his head. His stockings were flame embroidered with gold, and his black velvet shoes were decked with diamonds. M. le Duc came as a Greek in rich brocade and black velvet covered with French laces and embroidered with jewels of all colours. His cloak was of gold and silver French lace, bordered with Venetian lace, and edged with gems.

The Prince de Conti was another Persian, with a vest of black bordered with golden embroidery and bejewelled buttons. His caftan was blue covered with silver Spanish lace, and he wore a small turban of rich tissue of gold in flame, bedecked with chains of diamonds. His cloak was of Aurillac lace in gold and silver, lined with blue gauze brooched with gold. His brother the Prince de la Roche-sur-Yon had an outfit that was inventive rather than a national type. His flame velvet vest ended in four basques to form four compartments bordered with silver ornaments from which emerged a rose of diamonds. Between the compartments was a green lining sewn with little flowers in gold and silver, and he wore a half turban. The Comte de Vernandois was yet another Persian in cloth of gold, silver and flame. He vest was bordered with chains of diamonds, and all the buttonholes were outlined with gold embroidery and gems. His mantle was Spanish point lace in gold and silver, and his small turban was festooned with chains of jewels, and topped with plumes in flame and white.

Mlle de Blois, Françoise Marie, the youngest daughter of Louis XIV by Madame de Montespan, came as an Amazon. She wore a corselet of black velvet embroidered with gold and edged with chains of diamonds, from which hung a drapery in flame embroidered with silver. She wore slit sleeves, the lambrequins, copied from Roman armour, in black velvet, and a skirt of flame embroidered with gold and silver. Her helmet was of black velvet with veils of Aurillac lace falling down, and similar veils were suspended from her shoulders. Mlle de Nantes was a country girl in a bodice of gold brocade banded with black velvet, and decorated with gold and silver. She wore a transparent skirt of lace over another colour, and knots of gems where country girls put ribbons. The Duchesse de Nevers was a Moor in black velvet and flame, edged with gems and pearls. She wore a veil and a half turban·garnished with diamonds and pearls. Duchesse Sforce represented a nymph with masses of Spanish point lace in silver embroidered with gems, which had been designed by Montespan's sister Madame de Thianges. The Duchesse de Mortemar was a Persian, with a caftan of gold and cherry decked with silver Spanish point lace, and buttonholes of black velvet embroidered with gold and diamonds. Her vest was green covered with rich embroidery, and her mantle was a veil of Aurillac lace attached by knots of gems. She was Montespan's mother, and the family had benefited much from Athénaïs being the royal mistress. That very February the Marquis de Mortemar, son of Athénaïs Montespan's brother the Duc de Vivonne, married the third daughter of the minister Jean Baptiste Colbert. The bridegroom wore black velvet, which was usual, covered with black lace and flame-coloured ribbons, and the bride a black velvet gown

with a rich petticoat covered with gems and embroidery in gold and silver. Colbert married all his daughters into ducal houses.

Other guests at the king's masquerade were the Duc de Vendôme as a Bohemian, and M. de Soissons and the Chevalier de Savoye as Persians. M. le Grand was a Pole with a hat and border of marten's fur, and a black and gold caftan over a flame vest. The caftan had hanging sleeves and silver buttonholes. The Chevalier Colbert was an African with a vest of violet and gold, with hanging sleeves of Aurillac lace in gold and silver. He had a Moorish mask with great pearls at the ears, a collar, and a Moorish turban of gold and silver tissue, with plumes of flame and black, decorated with jewels. His mantle was French lace in gold and silver. The Marquis de Gesvres was another African, Comte de Castres a Persian. With the exceptions of the costume by Madame de Thianges, and the Duc de Villeroy who came as himself, all the costumes were designed by Jean Berain who had succeeded Henri Gissey as designer of the king's cabinet, and they were all made up by Jean Baraillon, tailor-in-ordinary to the king's ballet.[20]

There were other less formal masquerade parties like the Pulchinello Fair which the Marquise de Montespan held on 21 February 1685, where the stalls were all run by great ladies in masks. Carrousels were still held, although Louis now preferred to watch rather than to participate. In March 1685 the Marquis de Dangeau represented Charlemagne with five others all in black and gold, in quadrilles against the Saracens in green and gold. Another carrousel was held in May on the theme of the wars of Granada, the Spanish against the Moors. There was a presentation of the Four Seasons at Marly-de-Roi on 5 January 1686, when the Marquise de Montespan was Autumn, the Marquise de Maintenon was Winter, the Duc de Bourbon was Summer and his duchess Spring; their costumes were valued at 15,000 pistoles. Enjoyment became serious, however, when the princesses who were going to dance in *Le Bourgeois Gentilhomme* were told to take professional dancing lessons from the ballet masters Précourt and Farier from the Opéra.[21] The pattern was for endless balls, masquerades, banquets, comedies and carrousels at court for the winter and early spring, then the young noblemen left for the front to fight during the summer. Of course some entertainment continued at court during their absence, with parties in barges on the canals, outdoor dances in garden theatres, and visits to the different seats, but the greatest concentration of such activities was during the winter months, the Season. Once Louis XIV began to feel his years, the Dauphin and the grandchildren became the initiators of festivities, and the celebration continued. The glory of the king had to be illustrated in cloth of gold and silver, and chains of diamonds. It is a wonder the ostrich did not become extinct, the demands for its plumes were so great.

FOUR

Fashion
1680–1700

To Primi Visconti the surprising news in 1680 was the respect now shown at court to widow Scarron, the governess of Louis XIV's children by Montespan, who adored her more than their mother. A very devout woman who came from a Protestant family, the king had found her dull, but the more he saw her with his children, the more he came to appreciate that she had a sense of humour, and he purchased the estate of Maintenon which carried the rank of marquis, so that she could attend the court freely as Madame la Marquise de Maintenon. Montespan was behaving like a queen, sitting on armchairs and only offering princesses and duchesses stools although she was but a marquise. She spent about 800,000 francs a year on her clothes, jewels and potions, and was such a dominating character that in 1679 Louis XIV had turned his attention to a young girl of 18, whom her family had sent to court to exploit her looks, Marie Adelaide de Scorailles de Roussilhe. At Easter 1680 she was created Duchesse de Fontanges.[1] Montespan was incensed, and said it ruined the king's dress: 'To please his new divinity, the Monarch suddenly rejuvenated his attire. The most elegant stuffs became the substance of his garments, feathers reappeared. He joined to them emeralds and diamonds.'[2] He was 42, Montespan 44 and growing fat. Louis XIV had started to wear the fashionable mouse brown but in 1680 he went back to flame with everything, and made it the most fashionable tone for that year, as *Le Nouveau Mercure Galant* observed. Madame de Montespan put her finger on the point: he was trying to look younger, a dashing cavalier with baldrics and ribbons, plumes and gems. The Duchesse de Fontanges, by chance not design, affected fashion herself, and Montespan wrote:

At the chase one day, his nymph, whom nothing could stop, had her knot of riband caught and held by a branch; the royal lover compelled the branch to restore the knot, and went and offered it to his Amazon. Singular and sparkling, although lacking in intelligence, she carried herself this knot of riband to the top of her hair, and fixed it there with a long pin.

Fortune willed that this *coiffure*, without order or arrangement, suited her face, and suited it greatly. The King was the first to congratulate her on it; and all the courtiers applauded it, and this *coiffure* became the fashion of the day.

All the ladies, and the Queen herself, found themselves obliged to adopt it.[3]

Thanks to an inconvenient tree, ribbons in the hair *à la Fontanges* became the rage. It was ribbons that Fontanges named, not, as later writers have claimed, the entire headdress. The fashion came about by accident in the same way that Madame's falling off her horse in her German tippets made furs *à la palatine* the vogue. If the king approved, it was compulsory. That was all the young Duchesse de Fontanges was able to achieve. Her demise in 1681, some months after producing a son, was widely attributed to Madame de Montespan, who was said to have hired a pedlar Romani to take the young mistress poisoned gloves and fabrics.

A new official mistress was not appointed. Madame de Maintenon advised the king to think about the fate of his soul, and told him to treat the queen with more respect, which he did. This was just as well, for the

---

50 *Almanach Royal*, 1682, 'Bal à la Française'.
The vogue for lace sees women's caps returning to fashion, now competing with ribbons in the hair as launched by the Duchesse de Fontanges. A compromise will develop. The lean line of the 1670s is beginning to ease and women's waists are nearer the natural location. They all wear mantos, but cut off the shoulder slightly to display more of the neckline than the garment usually allowed, presumably to please Louis XIV. This was not enough – the *grand habit* was going to be completely off the shoulder. The man holding the music shows the bottom of his sleeve slashed open, a hint that sleeves will grow shorter on men's coats, which are highly embroidered.

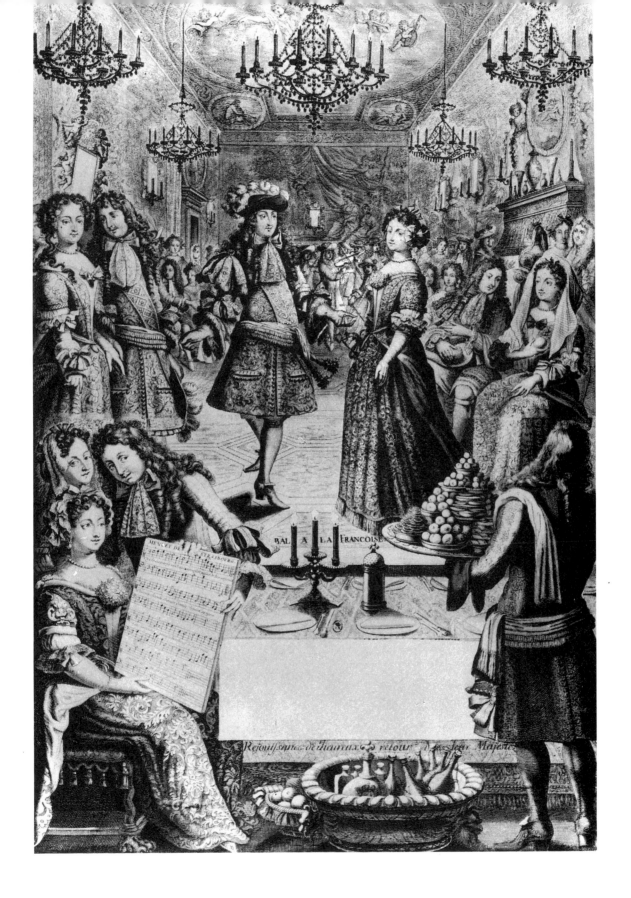

BAL A LA FRANCOISE.

MENUET DE STRASBOURG

Rejouissance de l'heureux retour de sa Majesté

queen Marie Thérèse was to die in 1683, after which, at an unknown date, Louis XIV married the drab, governessy, devout, Madame de Maintenon. She could not be queen as she was not of the blood royal and the Dauphin refused to recognise her as queen, a refusal he maintained for the remainder of his life, out of loyalty to his mother and her rank. A sober influence became established at court, which affected Louis XIV for the rest of his days.

Louis was still not interested in balancing the books, despite Colbert's efforts. A précis of his expenditure in 1680 shows:

Wars & extraordinaries	31,233,000 livres
King's household	9,184,000
Versailles, Marly and repairs to other seats	8,513,000
Queen's household	1,381,000
Monsieur's household	1,198,000
The Navy	4,928,000
Salaries and wages	2,302,000
Paris streets	58,000

Other costs: pensions, fortifications, repayments on debts, payments for secret service, roads, bridges, army depots etc.

Total royal expenditure	96,318,016
Total royal income	91,759,460[4]

The court had been frequently based at Versailles since 1672 but in 1682 the king considered the palace ready to accommodate the court and the government, Monsieur and Madame, and the Dauphin and his household. They all had to reside at Versailles henceforth, not at their own seats, and the ministers were not to reside in Paris. The king wanted business in the morning and hunting in the afternoon, and now he had both at Versailles; the enormous Louvre in Paris was left empty. The move was made on 6 March, with wagons stretching for miles, and in June 1682 a large number of Monsieur's homosexual entourage was banished from court. Louis had tolerated it while Monsieur had his own seat at Saint Cloud, because it kept his brother away from politics, but he did not want his clique at Versailles. Visconti remarked that there was an epidemic of disease among Monsieur's friends when the Marquis de La Vallière died in 1676. The marquis had made an advance to Visconti claiming that in Spain the monks were homosexual, in France the grandees, and in Italy everyone. Visconti had retorted that he was not and fled.[5]

Lavish display was still required for special occasions. The wedding of the Prince de Conti on 17 January 1680 saw the groom in an inestimably rich attire – a coat of black plush partitions on a straw ground, embroidered with great diamonds along the panels. The cloak was lined with black satin picked with diamonds. His sword was a marvel of diamond splendour. The straw was not a great success as a colour, Madame de Sevigné recorded. Other members of the Conti branch of the Bourbons, Monsieur le Duc, Madame la Duchesse and Mademoiselle de Bourbon all wore clothes covered with jewels, having three outfits for the three days of the ceremony.[6]

Elisabeth Charlotte's father Charles Louis Elector of the Rhineland Palatinate died in 1680, and her brother Charles in 1685. Louis XIV promptly claimed their lands in the name of Madame, regardless of the rights of the new Elector Neuburg. French troops occupied Strasbourg. Madame received a horrible example of how Louis XIV used marriages to justify his expansion, and now he was moving into Germany. Hitherto he had attacked Spain and the Netherlands, now the Rhineland was going to be ruined. In 1683 Louis XIV refused the Pope's request that he should help Vienna when she was being beseiged by the Turks. He was so intent on destroying Hapsburg power that he did not care if a new empire occupied eastern Europe and endangered Christianity. By 1686 feeling against France in Germany and Austria was so strong that the German princes, Austria and Spain formed the League of Augsburg against him. Louis XIV had razed Heidelburg Castle, Elisabeth Charlotte's home, to the ground, and seriously damaged the cathedrals of Manheim, Worms and Spiers. Europe was appalled. The man was a monstrous tyrant. Yet, even so, the hundreds of yards of best black velvet for the Elector's funeral were ordered from Lyons by special courier. In 1684 Aunt Sophia of Hanover married her daughter Sophia Charlotte, cousin to Elisabeth Charlotte, to Prince Frederick III of Brandenburg, and ordered the clothes from her agent Abbé Ballati in Paris. Sophia Charlotte wondered if she could wear a cloth of gold and silver gown with a petticoat in the same materials, and she wanted a gown in black velvet to show off her jewels. Aunt Sophia herself as a mature lady always wore black but supposed she would have to have a manto in brocade for the official entry into Berlin, possibly like the one the Princess of Friesland had in black and gold; she asked the abbé to decide, providing the outfit was not too gay. She was not sure if lavish embroidery was still in fashion and requested Ballati to find out. That September she wrote again to order four new suits for her husband Duke Ernst

August of Hanover, and four *grand habits* and four mantos for Sophia Charlotte, plus a fashion doll dressed in the latest style. These did not arrive in time for the wedding; Sophia was indignant that the tailors made her waists too big, and that there was no Spanish point lace on her black velvet. Notwithstanding such delays, Sophia and her son Prince George Louis, the future George I, escorted Sophia Charlotte to Berlin in November 1684, all attired in French finery. If politically the Germans detested Louis XIV, they could not resist the glamour of his court.[7]

In May 1685 the Doge of Genoa was required to travel to Versailles to bow before Louis XIV to apologize for annoying the French king. All Europe was expected to bend the knee before King Sun, and the feeling grew that this sun ought to be eclipsed. William of Orange was dedicated to doing precisely that.

In 1689 William and Mary II took Britain and the Netherlands into the League of Augsburg so that Louis XIV was now faced by an alliance of Austria, Spain, Sweden, Savoy, the German princes, Britain and the Netherlands. He did not have to worry to begin with, for as Sourches had noted in 1681 Louis had the biggest army in Europe, and a navy of 100–120 ships, the largest carrying 130 cannons. The alliance was not so well organized and suffered reversals to begin with but a Europe-wide resistance had started. Louis XIV was most gratified when the Siamese ambassador told him on 1 September 1686 that the two most magnificent courts in the whole world were those of the emperor of China and of the king of France, for Louis considered himself the equal of emperors.[8]

Finery was all very well for special occasions such as the reception of ambassadors, but the unofficial queen Madame de Maintenon persuaded Louis to dress with greater sobriety. The trend towards browns was given new encouragement, and for the rest of his reign Louis XIV now wore brown suits, and only donned bejewelled outfits for weddings, birthdays and such. This was the sort of king whom Saint Simon first saw in 1691:

He was always dressed in brownish colours with a light embroidery, never on the skirts, sometimes nothing except gold buttons, sometimes black velvet. The waistcoat was always cloth or satin in red, blue, green heavily embroidered. Never any rings, or jewels except on his shoe buckles and garters, and the hat always bordered with Spanish point lace with a white plume. He always wore the blue sash [of the order of the Holy Ghost] under his coat except for wed-

dings or other similar festivities when he wore it on top, very long, with eight or ten millions in jewels. Heavy scents gave him headaches, so he only allowed orange flower water.

This was a total contrast to the flamboyant Louis of the 1660s with his fondness for flame, frills and diamonds every day. Madame Elisabeth Charlotte said it was due to the influence of that 'drab', as she called her, the new Marquise de Maintenon.

Madame's husband was as a great a contrast as could be. Saint Simon described Monsieur:

He was a little pot-bellied man, mounted upon a scaffold his shoe heels were so high, always dressed up like a woman, covered with rings, bracelets, jewels everywhere, with a long *perruque* displayed in front, in black and powdered and ribbons everywhere it was possible to put them, drenched in all sorts of perfumes and the height of cleanliness. He was accused of wearing a hint of rouge; the nose very long, a beautiful mouth and eyes, the face full but very long.[9]

Maintenon was not going to have any effect on Monsieur Philippe, and Elisabeth Charlotte had stopped trying. She bore him three children of whom two survived, and thereafter they slept apart. His daughters wore father's jewels far more than mother's.

The lean line of the 1670s overlapped into the 1680s, and it was 1682 before a new trend could be discerned. Men's sleeves began to open up, with either the bottom part of the seam of the sleeve left undone, so that it could be turned up, or else in a buttoned sleeve which could be undone, and turned back to form large cuffs near the elbow. These indicated that sleeves were going to grow shorter, and by 1686 the shorter sleeve for men was established with very large cuffs just below the elbow called spaniels' ears. The ladies had had short sleeves since 1670, so the men had taken time to catch up. The tightness relaxed into an easier silhouette, sleeves were a little wider, the waist looser, and the coat skirts a little fuller, as an easier air came into fashion. Cravats became more noticeable. In 1678 one ribbon was thought sufficient to ornament a cravat in front. By 1686 it had become six ribbons and more in red satin crowded underneath the cravat. Ribbons were making a comeback and were to sprout on the cuffs, on the shoulder, on the sword hilt, and on the hat. After all the Dauphin was in his twenties, and if the court was growing sober, outside in the town fashion could be fun. Monseigneur Louis began by being very vain about his blond curls, and like his father did not adopt a periwig for some time. He had inherited his curls from both his parents, and not until 1686 did the

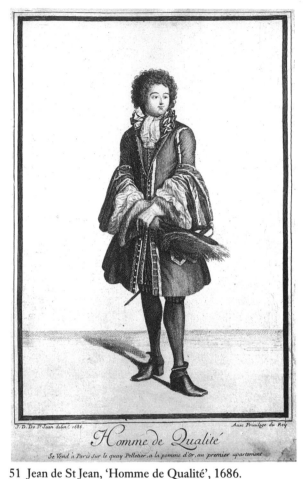

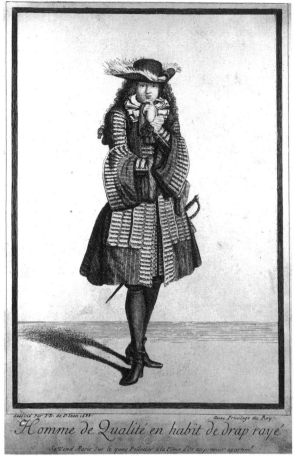

51 Jean de St Jean, 'Homme de Qualité', 1686.
The short sleeve with large spaniels' ears' cuffs is established. Stripes have become the dominant pattern, and four vertical pockets the norm. The number of ribbons behind the cravat has increased to almost a dozen, and fringed gloves are in fashion. The knee roll has commenced life as a feature. The length of the coat and vest are completely in the style of the English establishment. The man does not appear to be wearing a wig, but neither did the Dauphin up to this particular year, 1686. (*Victoria and Albert Museum, London*)

52 Jean de St Jean, 'Homme de Qualité en habit de drap rayé, 1688.
This suit is in a striped fabric decked heavily with braid. The new feature is that the vest sleeves have outgrown the coat sleeves, and this was the chief style for 1688–91. The four vertical pockets remain standard in this decade. Hats could still be cocked any way the wearer pleased. (*Victoria and Albert Museum, London*)

Dauphin decide that long hair was a nuisance when hunting, and that he would go over to wigs, although he always had them made blond, whereas his father usually wore black wigs now. This convertion ensured the continuance of perruques into the next century. When the heir took up a style it had some significance. Periwigmakers responded by piling on even more hair, and perruques grew both upwards and downwards like a mane of leonine splendour. As Vanbrugh's Lord Foppington put it in *The Relapse* (Act I sc.iii): 'a perwig to a man should be like a mask

to a woman: nothing should be seen but his eyes.' His wig had 20 ounces of hair in it.

In December 1684 *Le Nouveau Mercure Galant* said that four pockets on the coat were now essential. Hitherto in the 1660s and '70s pockets had been simple horizontal slits and no more, but the 1680s decided to make them a feature. Four vertical pockets, outlined with braid or buttons, became the dominant type for that decade. Louis XIV wore them, Jean Dieu de St Jean engraved prints of them, and they spread across Europe as the standard type. There also grew, however, a sub-fashion of about 1686–91 in the form of a vogue for bizarre pockets. Only two of these were

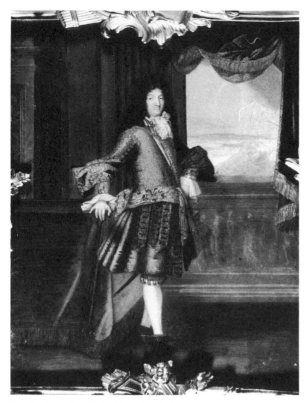

53 Petitot, 'Louis XIV', *c.* 1688/9.
The king is shown in the very latest style with the longer vest sleeves, the four vertical pockets, and the increasing pleating in coat skirts as the back view is now in vogue. The suit shows the impact of Madame de Maintenon for it is plain cloth, with no embroidery, in a sober tone, and the decoration is restricted to buttons and buttonholes. Only the embroidered sash and the cravat ribbons show some of the colourful character that used to typify Louis XIV. (*Formerly at Mentmore, Bucks*)

long, so that they showed below the cuff, and concealed the shirt sleeve completely. It was clear that now the English three-piece suit had became an institution, French tailors were looking for ways to give it seasonal changes and variations to keep the market lively. No customer must be allowed to think that having bought a suit he was dressed for life; sleeves, pockets, skirts, must all be changed to oblige the customer to buy another one for fear of being out of date. The composition did not alter; it was set for centuries with a coat, a waistcoat and kneebreeches, later trousers. Variation could not enter by

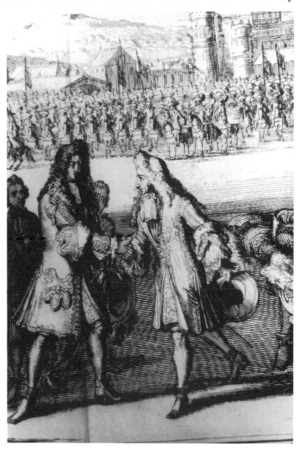

54 Romain de Hooghe, 'Louis XIV [left] Receiving James II into Exile at Saint Germain en Laye', 1688.
A relief from vertical pockets were the bizarre pockets, a sub-fashion between 1686 and 1691. This example has affected the cuff too, and allowed for a little fantasy on suits, now that they were an institution. It appears to have been inspired by a butterfly, but other examples were geometric. Catholic James II had to flee from England when Parliament invited his Protestant daughter Mary II and her Dutch husband to replace him. It was the defeat of Louis XIV's scheme to impose a Catholic regime on Britain.

worn at a time and they were horizontal not vertical, but they allowed for fantastic variations as a relief, perhaps, from four pockets of rigid verticality. The shape was full of variety with pocket flaps like butterfly wings, curves, hexagons, zigzags and triangles, and Louis XIV wore them too. Thus between 1684 and 1691 pockets vertical and bizarre enjoyed an importance that they have not had since. In the 1690s pockets settled back to being a plain component of the suit, with just two horizontal ones with a flap *à la maréchal*, for they resembled the flaps of a marshall's portfolio.

Sleeves began to change again in 1688. Vests or waistcoats had long sleeves, so when coat sleeves were shortened vest sleeves had to be too; but by this date men began to wear the vest sleeves unaltered and

55 Male dummy figure, *c.* 1690/1.
Over 1690–1 the difference between coat and vest
sleeves was 'corrected', so that they became equal
in length. The four vertical pockets and the mass
of ribbon behind the cravat overlapped the decade
into the 1690s. Periwigs were growing upwards
and downwards in a vain effort to match the
soaring heights of women's commodes, and
increasingly resembled a lion's mane. The fabric
is plain, as stripes start to go out of fashion, but his
waistcoat is rich. (*Victoria and Albert Museum,*
London)

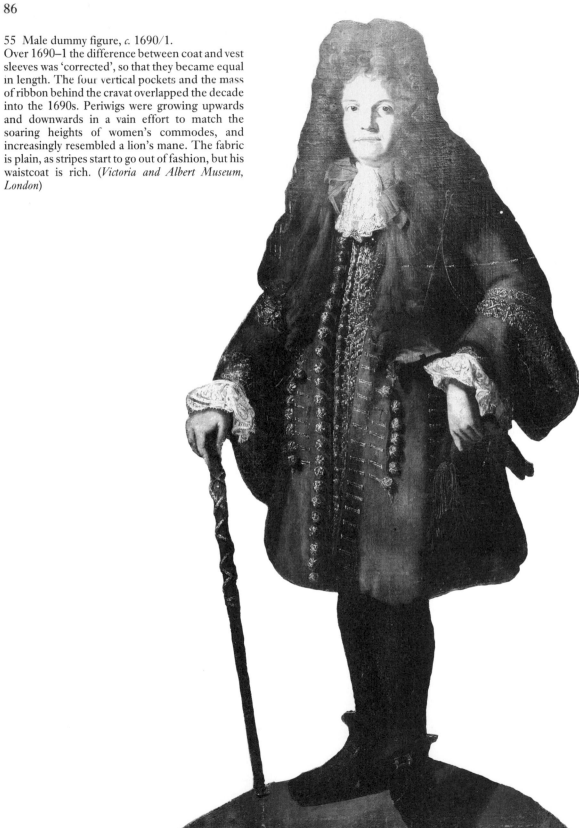

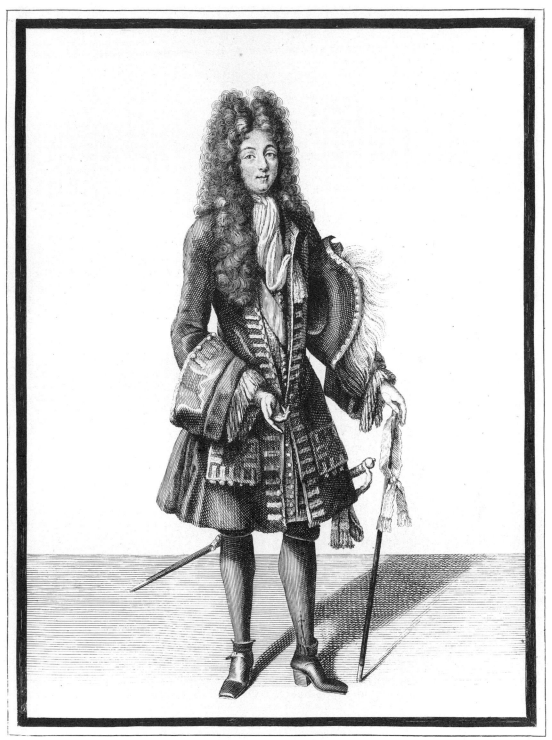

56 André Trouvain, 'Monsieur le Prince de Conty', 1694.
In 1692 the steinkerque cravat knocked ribbons out of
vogue, and brought an informal air into fashion to contrast
with the formal suits, wigs, fringed gloves, canes, swords,
and plumed hats. Clocked stockings are coming into favour,
and the knee roll grows larger. Pockets *à la maréchale* oust
vertical ones. The coat is trimmed with braid, but not
covered with it, for that would resemble liveries.
(*Stadtmuseum, Munich*)

introducing a new garment into the suit, so it was the detail that had to be altered. Consequently the design of menswear became more sophisticated. It was no longer a question of big cloaks, small capes, doublets or cassocks succeeding each other in and out of fashion. Now it was suits on a permanent basis, so the fashionable changes had to work within a new discipline, and change the pockets, sleeves, or cravat, but not the whole structure. The uniform for men had arrived.

Lengthening the vest sleeve was only a prelude to lengthening the coat sleeve, so after about three years of imbalance the two were harmonized in 1691/2. The overall trend in men's clothes in this decade was towards a grand sobriety in keeping with Louis XIV's more respectable image. Ribbons were cleared away in favour of a plain cravat and less fussy silhouette. Decoration was restricted to braid down the seams and centre front, and on the spaniels' ears cuffs. While men had been free to cock their hats in any way they liked, and Louis XIV had preferred the military type cocked up in front when riding, by 1693 the first examples of the geometric cock appeared, where the hat was turned up on three sides in equal proportion like a triangle. For a time it had to co-exist with hats cocked in all directions, but after 1700 the geometrical cock became the standard type for the next century, as the three-cornerd or tricorne hat. It was a hint of the Age of Reason ahead with its fondness for order, balance, proportion, as a change from Baroque grandeur and rhythm.

Accident and chance could set off a masculine fashion as much as a feminine one. At the battle of Steinkirk on 3 August 1692 the Anglo-Dutch army, under William III, was so uncivilized as to attack the French army, under Maréchal de Luxembourg, at dawn before the marshall and the French officers had finished dressing. They were obliged to dash out and fight before they had time to tie their cravats, so they twisted them out of the way and stuck the end through a buttonhole. The steinkerque was born, and since the French managed to win the battle despite the distress of having to fight in imperfect dress, the steinkerque cravat was quickly taken up by the court as a symbol of national success. The correct buttonhole to push the end through became established as the second one from the top. There was such a craze for steinkerques that women adopted them too but as they lacked buttonholes on their mantos, they pinned the ends to the rever. It was however a *habit de ville*, a town fashion, so it could not

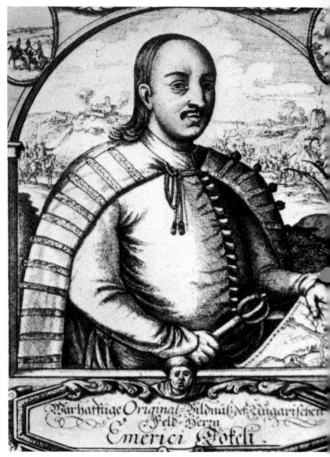

57 Anon., 'Emeric Thököly Prince of Transylvania', *c.* 1690.
Thököly wore his cloak or *mente* with the revers braided back and held by buttons all the way down, possibly to give his arms greater freedom. This distinctive style was probably reported to his ally Louis XIV, for the French court launched a version of Thököly's style in 1694. Thököly was leader of the Hungarian Reformed Church against Catholic Austria. (*Hungarian National Museum, Budapest*)

be worn at Versailles where the plain lace cravat worn straight was still required. Even so, steinkerques lasted into the 1720s.

A fashion moving in the opposite direction, from civilians to the army appeared in 1694. Louis XIV seems to have wished to commemorate an ally, for the *habit de Teckeli* was launched. John Evelyn had noted in 1690 the success that Count Teckeli was having in Transylvania, so the name was known as far away as England. Teckeli was the western version of the Hungarian name Thököly. Count Emeric Thököly was leader of the Hungarian Protestants against

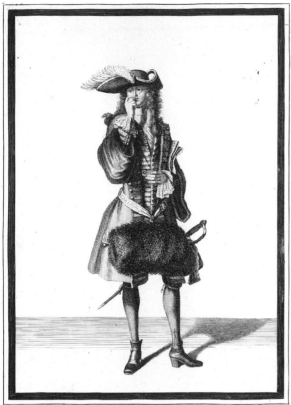

Homme de qualité en habit de Teckeli

se vend à Paris sur le Quay Pelletier à la pomme d'or au premier appartement

58 Jean de St Jean, 'Homme de Qualité en habit de Teckeli', 1694.
The buttoned-down revers are transferred to the coat, and given a contrast facing. Many armies adopted the concept in the next century. Obviously there is a difference in applying Thököly's look to coats, when he wore it on a cloak, but in France cloaks were out of fashion, and coats and overcoats were in. Muffs have become enormous, and cocking the hat was still a matter of personal taste. Shoe buckles ousted bows about 1678 and thereafter shoes were plain. The block heel was probably the sort devised by Monsieur in 1661, for they had been slimmer before then. (*Victoria and Albert Museum, London*)

Catholic Austria, which was trying to suppress the Hungarian Reformed Church. As Louis XIV wished to undermine Austria he encouraged Thököly and became his ally. The Turks helped him too, and in 1690 the Sultan appointed Thököly Prince of Transylvania. Thököly was known for wearing the *mente* over his dolman with the revers fastened back all the way down the front with braid and buttons, and it was this feature which was translated to the western

coat. Buttoned-back revers, showing a contrast lining, were considered very smart by the military, and in the eighteenth century many armies adopted Thököly's style on their uniforms: so the Hungarian's influence was considerable, helped of course by the French engravings of the style.

Thököly also wore Turkish caftans at his court, for the Sultan had the oriental custom of presenting caftans to favoured persons. Marco Polo had noted the same custom in China under Kublai Khan, so it was long established. Thököly presented caftans in turn, and so was instrumental in aiding the adoption of Turkish garments in Hungary. In January 1687 the Dauphin at Versailles had received two very rich caftans from the Sultan, one embroidered in gold, the other in silver, so when he wanted to appear as a Turk at a masquerade he had the correct garments.[10]

An even more exotic fashion affected menswear from about 1697: the sleeves *à la pagode*. Whether they were copied from an actual pagoda, or inspired from prints of pagodas, is not certain, but the shape of the Chinese tower, narrow at the top and wide at the bottom, was applied to sleeves. This resulted in the cuff and mouth of the sleeve being very wide, and the sleeve head very narrow. Such very full sleeves remained in fashion for the next 20 years. They were a forerunner of the craze for chinoiserie in the eighteenth century, and reflected the impact of the East India Companies' imports.

After 1683, fashion for the ladies became as established as the suit for men. It was the *grand habit* with its boned bodice for court, with the regulations over trains – 11 ells for a queen, 9 ells for a king's daughter, 7 ells for a king's granddaughter, 5 ells for a princess of the blood, and 3 ells for a duchess. Everywhere else the manto reigned supreme: at the theatre, at dances, at dinners, at promenades, and as seen already Sophia of Hanover considered it suitable for her official entry into Berlin. In England Princess Anne still had some doubts, for she wrote from Windsor Castle on 20 October 1696 to query whether mantos, would be suitable for William III's birthday ball. Lady Fitzhardinge thought not, saying a full-boned gown like the *grand habit* would be better, while mantos would be acceptable at the playhouse. In the event William III raised no objections to mantos so Princess Anne wore one to his ball.[11] Mary II, William's wife and co-monarch, had died the year before, so her sister Anne was now first lady. Mary had been a keen wearer of mantos herself. They were more comfortable than boned bodices, and they were

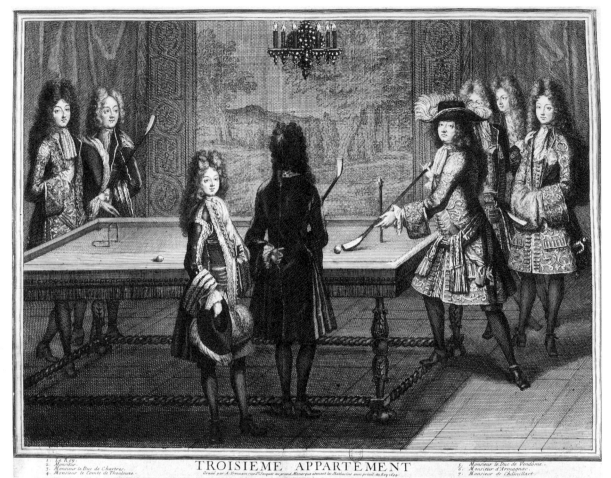

TROISIEME APPARTEMENT

1. Le Roy.
2. Monsieur.
3. Monsieur le Duc de Chartres.
4. Monsieur le Comte de Thoulouse.

5. Monsieur le Duc de Vendôme.
6. Monsieur d'Armagnac.
7. Monsieur de Chamillart.

Gravé par A. Trouvain rue S.t Jacque au grand Monarque venant des Mathurins avec privil. du Roy 1694.

warmer for they covered the shoulders, whereas exposed shoulders and necks had dominated women's fashions since the 1650s until the welcome arrival of mantos in the 1670s. Louis XIV might find it difficult to understand their popularity, and the mantos' refusal to disappear at his command, but he was going to find that where women's fashion was concerned, the only official opposition inside France was women's obstinate sporting of what they liked to wear. Here his abolute majesty the King Sun was ignored. Mantos outlived him.

The craze for ribbons reawakened by the Duchesse de Fontanges affected clothes, and they tumbled down the front of the stomacher on the manto, in rows of bows. Ribbons blossomed on parasols, on necklaces and fans, but they tended to be restricted to the upper half of the body. Bows did not adorn petticoats where braid and lace remained the chief ornaments until 1685, when fringed petticoats began to appear with between three and nine rows of fringes.

59 André Trouvain, 'Troisième Appartement', 1694.
Louis XIV playing billiards with his brother Monsieur, who stands at the far left of the table looking impossibly young for 54, and wearing a highly embroidered coat. His son Philippe Duc de Chartres stands on the far right with a muff and steinkerque cravat. Etiquette required males to be uncovered in the presence whereas the king kept his hat on, so Louis plays covered. His highly patterned coat still carries the baldric and sash of the 1670s, but the younger generation has discarded them. Sleeves have become narrow again as in the 1670s but a change is about to occur. The boy is the bastard Comte de Toulouse. (*Bibliothèque Nationale, Paris*)

Some ladies combined all three, so that a petticoat could have braid, lace and fringes alternating in rows. The vogue for ribbons made its biggest impact on the cap. At first it had seemed that ribbons in the hair *à la Fontanges* would end the popularity of lace pinners and the return to laced caps, but by 1683 bows of ribbons were being applied to caps. A compromise was

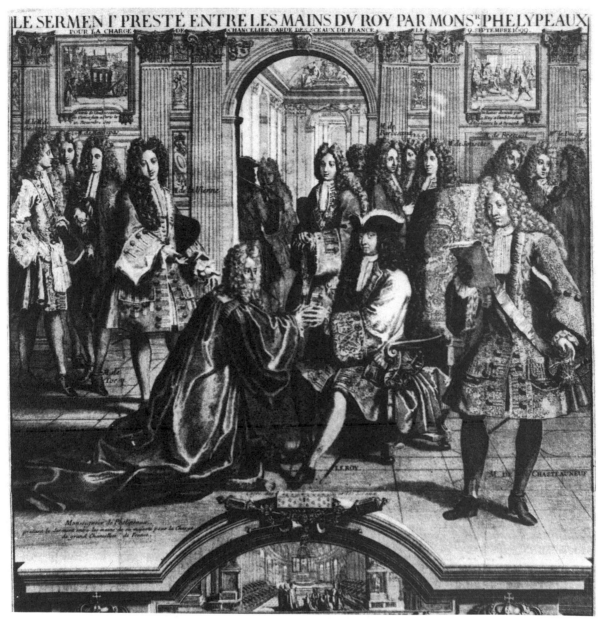

LE SERMEN T PRESTÉ ENTRE LES MAINS DV ROY PAR MONS^R PHELYPEAUX

achieved whereby the hair in front was dressed upwards with ribbons *à la Fontanges*, and the cap or pinners behind it could remain in place. The chief characteristic of the Fontanges hairstyle was height; she had tied her hair up with ribbon. Thus to keep in proportion the frill on the cap had to grow taller, both to support the hair and to harmonize with its height. We do not know who had the idea of applying the Fontanges bows to the back of the cap, but this is where the Fontanges ribbons came to be fixed. The cap in France was called a commode, not a fontange,

60 Anon., 'Monsr. Phelypeaux Takes the Oath as Chancellor and Keeper of the Seals, 9 September 1699. The pagoda sleeve takes over, initially growing as wide as cuffs. Then the cuffs are enlarged so the sleeve grows even wider, but remains narrow at the top like a Chinese pagoda. This sleeve lasted a decade into the next century before a modification developed. Coat skirts are wider to echo the bustles worn by women, and very full in the back. As this is a formal occasion, steinkerque cravats may not be worn. Clocked stockings are still in vogue. (*Author's photograph*)

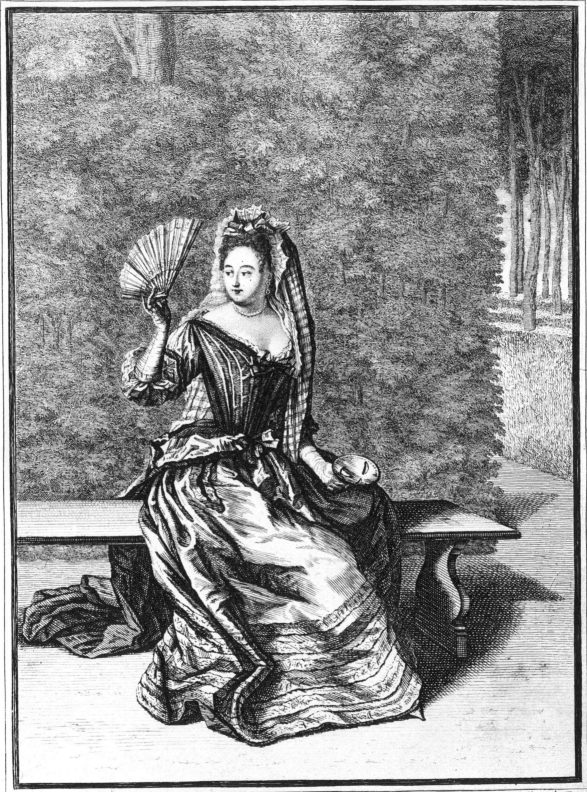

J.D. De St. Jean delin 1686   Auec Priuilege du Roy

Femme de Qualité aux Thuilleries

Se Vend A Paris Sur le quay Pelletier, a la pomme d'Or, au premier apartement which referred to a ribbon on the cap.

Madame agreed with her German relations in June 1687 that by now all the women, from little girls to the over-eighties, were wearing ribbon coiffures, that is hair dressed with ribbons backed by a ribbon-decked commode cap. The young had them in bright colours, the older in dark or black, but Madame was resisting the new fashion. She found the rustling of the ribbons too noisy, and she did not like the way the hair was scraped up off the face, exposing the ears, which some women were now painting white. Of course at Versailles no caps were permitted with the *grand habit*, Madame's usual indoor attire, so she did not have to adopt them.[12]

The vocabulary of the new style became elaborate. Originally commode had meant the wire frame which was developed to support the cap frill, but it became the term for the cap too. Where a cap was draped with lace pinners it was a *frelange*. The hair brushed up in front had to be supported, so it was given a wire called a palisade, and the style was dubbed a *tour* or tower. The English adopted all the French terms, and in 1685 Mary Evelyn wrote her *Fop's Dictionary* to explain the vocabulary. Her father John Evelyn published it in 1690 as *Mundus Muliebris*. She makes it clear that the fontange was the top knot or bow, and that on the back of the commode cap the fontange bow was placed over the duchesse bow. In the early 1680s *fontange* and *duchesse* meant bows of ribbon in the hair; by the middle of the decade they were ribbons on the back of the cap. A knot in the hair which tied the curls together was termed a *meutrière*, murderer, and a little bow peeping out between the pinner and the cap was a *sorti*. To give extra height artificial hair pieces were devised called *tours*, but eventually this word was used for the whole structure. Curls on the forehead were *favourites*. As the commode could not be worn with the *grand habit*, the hair was decorated instead with

diamond pins and other gems stuck into the tower like stars and called a firmament.[13]

Madame might not care for the new style but Mary II liked it and considered a commode headdress and a manto *à la sultane* (fastened with loops and brooches) appropriate dress for her official arrival in London in 1688 when Parliament invited her to replace her Catholic father James II. As a result she towered over her husband William III, which was why several men, including Louis XIV, began to object to this soaring spire of lace, wire, ribbons, and hair; it made them look small. Periwigs were increased in height, but they never managed to rise to the same dominance as the ladies' commode for they did not employ wired lace to extend the hair.

Louis XIV had an amusing story about the style, which Madame promptly explained in a letter to Aunt Sophia in Hanover on 26 January 1688: 'The King told us at table today about a hairdresser called Allart, who dressed the ladies' heads so high in England, that they could not get into their Sedan chairs, so they have had to have their Chairs made higher in order to permit them to follow the French fashion.'[14] Certain doors would have needed adjustment too. Louis XIV said it was a very inconvenient fashion, but no one listened, so he had to repeat his criticism until in 1691 his illegitimate daughters obliged by reducing their commodes to two tiers. This was copied briefly, but by 1693 three and four tiers were back again, and the king's objections made no real impact. Women wore commodes in the grounds at Versailles, at the other seats, and even Madame came round to wearing some black ribbons and lace on her head as it looked too singular to be without.

Madame felt like wearing all black in 1692, when Louis XIV told Monsieur he wanted his son Philippe Duc de Chartres to marry Louis's illegitimate daughter by Montespan, Mademoiselle de Blois. Madame told her son to refuse! Marry a bastard indeed, when she was descended from kings of England and Scotland and electors of the Rhineland Palatinate! Young Philippe, only 17, said he would obey his mother, but when he was summoned to an audience with the king, was too scared to say no. Madame was so furious she slapped her son's face in public, and Monsieur received the biggest dressing down of his life for giving in to his brother's proposal. Saint Simon said Madame looked like Ceres after the rape of Proserpine by Pluto. Madame lost this round, but she drummed it into her son's head to guard himself against the scheming of the royal bastards. He

61 Jean de St Jean, 'Femme de Qualité aux Thuilleries', 1686.
This lady wears a manto with the skirt pushed right back into a narrow train, so that the petticoat is given greater prominence. The period's craze for stripes can be seen in the braided rows all round the petticoat, and not simply in front as previously. Cutting the manto back at the neck was only a brief vogue over 1682–6, thereafter the covered up character returned. Her hair is tied up with bows in the manner of the Duchesse de Fontanges and over it she wears several layers of pinners. A frill has started to sprout at the top and this feature is about to be taken to its extreme. (*Victoria and Albert Museum, London*)

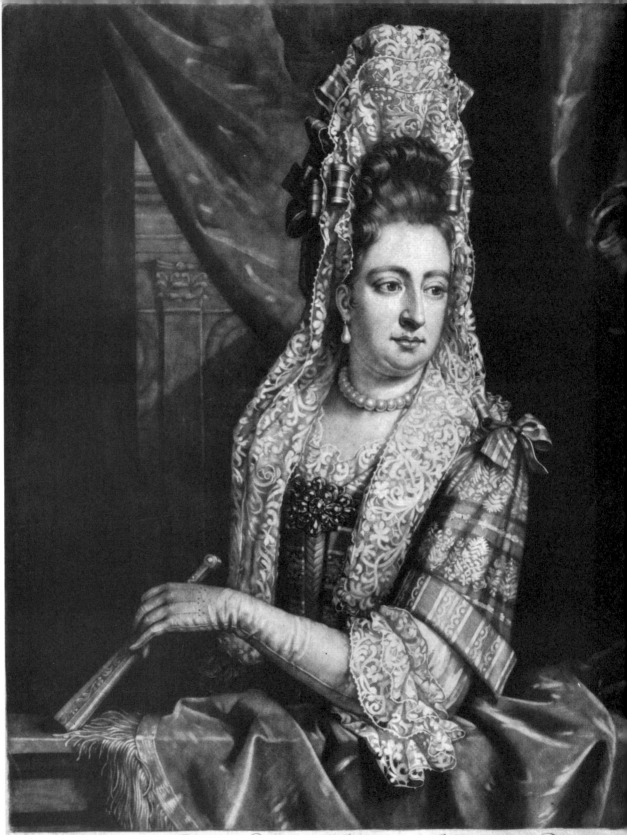

Maria D.G. Angliæ Scotiæ Franciæ et Hiberniæ Regina.

Vanderva... Pinxit   J. Smith fecit   Cum Privilegio Regis   Sold by E. Cooper at ÿ 3 Pidgeons in Bedford Street.

was the king's legitimate nephew, and should take precedence over bastards. This lessson did sink in and young Philippe was to emerge later as the bastards' chief opponent. Madame's pride was soothed somewhat by the good news from Hanover. The emperor in Vienna had promoted Ernst August from duke to elector, so Aunt Sophia was now an electress. Their minister Grote was sent to Vienna to collect the documents and there had to wear Spanish court dress, the black doublet and kneebreeches with the stiff golilla collar. In March 1693 the electoral bonnet arrived, so the family ordered ermine mantles. Even better news lay ahead, for in January 1701 Frederick William III of Brandenburg was crowned first king of Prussia, so Aunt Sophia's daughter Sophia Charlotte was crowned queen. She wore a dress of cloth of gold with diamonds down the seams, and a purple train embroidered with golden crowns and eagles. Madame Elisabeth Charlotte could hold up her head again.[15]

The struggle between Louis XIV and the Hapsburgs of Vienna over Spain was entering a vicious phase. Monsieur's daughter Queen Marie Louise of Spain was poisoned in 1689. The Hapsburgs were out to counter the French connection, and poor Carlos II was given a Hapsburg bride who proved to be so bossy that Carlos preferred the company of the French ambassador, who of course was all sympathy and compassion. The daggers were out. Another war loomed.

The decoration of the exposed petticoat was an important feature of the fashion for mantos. While petticoats in the 1660s and '70s had been ornamented with braid of gold or silver down the front and around the hem, it was not until the 1680s that all-over decoration became the vogue. As more of the petticoat had to be displayed, the gown was pulled back further until it was no more than a train at the back. Striped fabrics were the dominant pattern in the 1680s so striped petticoats visible all the way round became a

characteristic of the period. By the 1690s the train was making a comeback from being banished so far round to the rear, had regained the sides of the lady, and was being decorated itself. Lace, frills, fringes, braid were now added to the train to give it more importance, and the view of a lady from behind was given more consideration. This ornamentation needed some support so *culs de crin*, horsehair bottoms, were devised and the silhouette from about 1693 became a bustle and a cascading train. As bustles sway when the wearer is walking, causing the train to tremble and swing, women were given a new device with which to charm men, and to make an effective exit. The look was growing more sophisticated after the bold stripes of the 1680s. The stripes were interset with flowers, and three rows of decoration on the petticoats replaced nine. The commode headdress began to taper more, and the size of the bows was considerably reduced. The stomacher became a piece of brocade without any bows down the front, as an element of restraint entered women's fashion, to accord with the greater sense of sober grandeur at Versailles now that Madame de Maintenon determined the king's wardrobe.

Louis XIV was eager to detach Savoy from the League of Augsburg. After all, France had married his Aunt Chrétienne and Monsieur's other daughter by Henriette Anne, Anne Marie, to dukes of Savoy, so what was the country doing siding with his enemies? He offered an enormous bribe, the marriage of the duke's daughter to the future king of France no less, the Dauphin's eldest son Louis Duc de Bourgogne. Savoy had already suffered from French troops swarming across the country and occupying the foothills, so the duke Victor Amadeus II was not in a position to refuse. In addition Louis XIV offered him the address of royal highness. The prospective bride aged 11, Marie Adelaide of Savoy, was the eldest child of the duke and Anne Marie d'Orléans, so she was Monsieur's granddaughter. Anne Marie was only one when her mother Henriette Anne had died, so she was brought up alongside her sister Marie Louise by their young stepmother the second Madame Elisabeth Charlotte, who taught them the importance of morality, principle and rank. When the girls left Versailles, Marie Louise to Spain in 1679, and Anne Marie to Savoy in 1685, Elisabeth Charlotte wrote to them several times a week about events at Versailles and advising them on conduct, so when Anne Marie bore Marie Adelaide she was able to pass on much information about the splendid court of Louis XIV.

---

62 J. Smith after VanderVaart, 'Mary II Queen Regnant of the United Kingdoms, and of her New England Colonies', 1688.
The cap zooms upwards. The frills are built with wire commodes, and draped with gros point lace pinners to constitute a frelange. The hair is swept *en tour*. The bows at the back are the fontanges and the duchesse. The manto covers the shoulders and is always laced in front. Its pattern of stripes is interset with flowers, showing the less rigid designs to come. The shift is edged with gros point lace. (*Victoria and Albert Museum, London*)

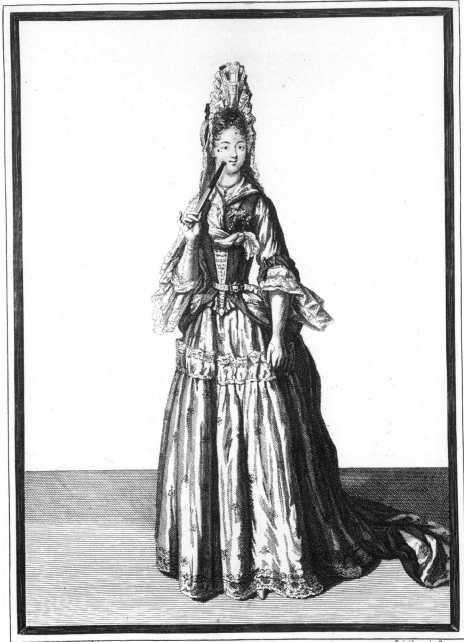

dessiné par I. D. De S. Iean 1693.   auec Priuilege du Roy

Femme de qualité en Stenkerke et falbala

se vend a Paris sur le Quay Pelletier a la Pomme d'Or au premier appartement

63 Jean de St Jean, 'Femme de Qualité en Stenkerke et falbala', 1693.

This manto has a contrast lining, which shows at the revers and cuffs, and in the turn back sides of the train. She imitates the male steinkerque cravat but has to pin it to the rever as women lacked buttonholes, except on their riding habits. The frill on the petticoat, the falbala, was a simple style in the midst of skirts covered in rows of fringe and lace. In 1691 Louis XIV wished that commode headdress would diminish. They did not but they grew narrower to taper more like a spire. Gloves and fans remain essential accessories. (*Victoria and Albert Museum, London*)

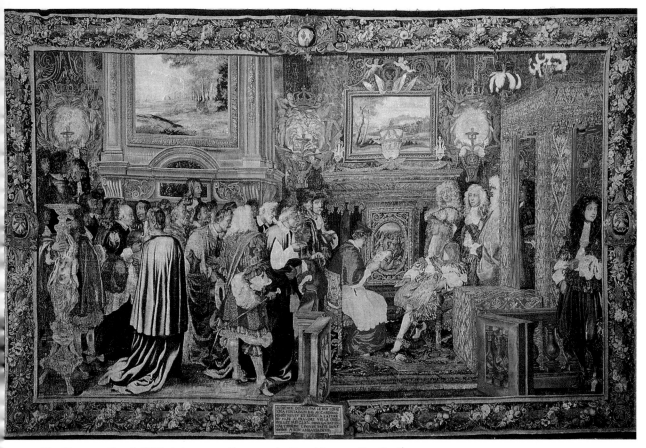

Versailles Tapestry, 'Louis XIV giving an audience to the Papal Legate, Cardinal Chigi, at Fontainebleau on 29 July 1664'.

Relations between Louis XIV and the Pope were often strained. Here the audience takes place behind the balustrade around the state bed. Louis wears a pale pink suit with a short doublet and wide kneebreeches decked with silver ribbons at the elbows, waist and knees. His dark blond hair made blond wigs fashionable at court in this decade. One courtier with his back to the spectator is wearing the new coat. The high-heeled shoes of French style have wired bows, and the wide lace collars are about to be replaced by cravats. *(Musée de Versailles, cliché des Musées Nationaux)*

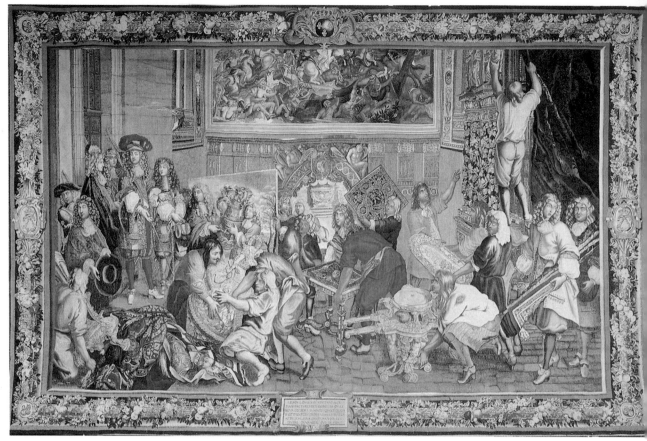

2 Atelier Le Blond, Versailles Tapestry, 'Visit of Louis XIV to the Manufactory at
Gobelins on 15 October 1667'.
1667 was the year Louis XIV tried out the English look of a long coat and waistcoat,
with narrower breeches, here in his favourite colour, flame red, embroidered with
gold. His little brother Monsieur Philippe, Duc d'Orléans is to the right of the
king, and Charles Le Brun, director of the manufactory, with his hat in his hand,
supervises the display of its products: tapestries, carpets, textiles, furniture in silver
and inlaid woods, ornaments, silver plate, pictures, and sculptures. Versailles was a
showplace for French products to impress the world. *(Musée de Versailles, cliché des
Musées Nationaux)*

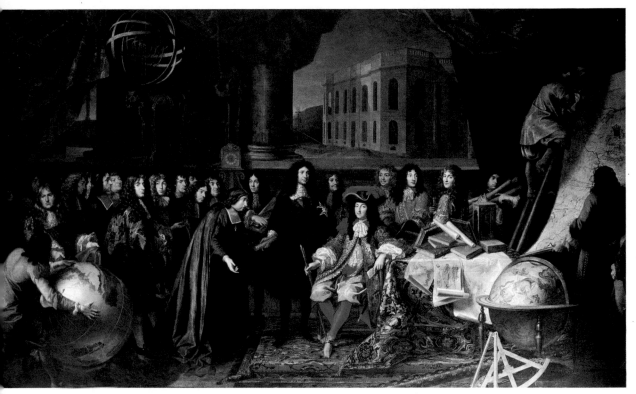

Henri Testelin, 'Louis XIV establishing the Academy of Sciences (1666) and the Observatory (1667)'.
Louis XIV is decked with flame ostrich plumes, flame ribbons and flame stockings. His coat and vest are covered with floral embroidery in many colours, while his breeches are decorated with gold galloon. He has changed over to the cravat, and his sleeves show the beginnings of descent towards the wrist. Beside the king stands a secretary of state in ministerial black. Louis XIV encouraged the arts and the sciences, in order to add to his glory. *(Musée de Versailles, cliché des Musées Nationaux)*

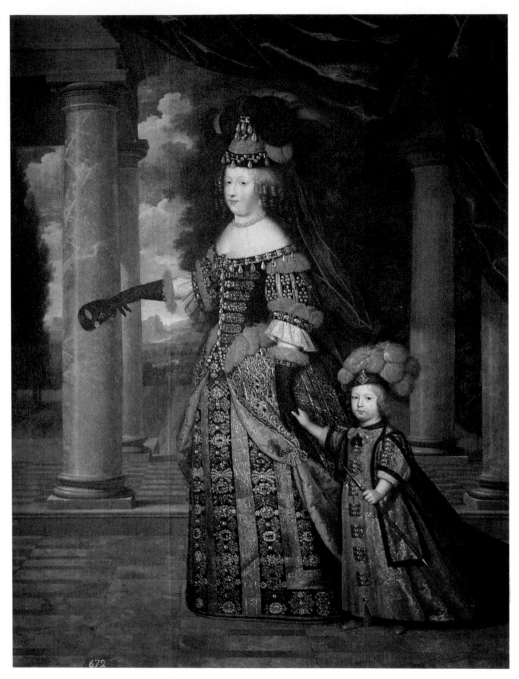

4 Pierre Mignard, 'Queen Marie Thérèse and the Dauphin Louis in masquerade costume', 1665.

The queen wears a fashionable dress of black velvet, heavily embroidered with silver, and lined with flame-coloured silk brocaded with silver. Droplet pearls edge the corsage and the front of the bodice. The petticoat is covered with some of the Crown jewels, sapphires and rubies in pearl settings, pearl and gold and silver brooches and diamond clusters, set between strips of gold galloon. The Dauphin is a huntsman with his axe, in a Turkish-style caftan of cloth of gold, with a cloth of silver cloak, fastened with silver frogging and pearls. Ostrich plumes were a mark of distinction, and were expensive. *(Museo del Prado)*

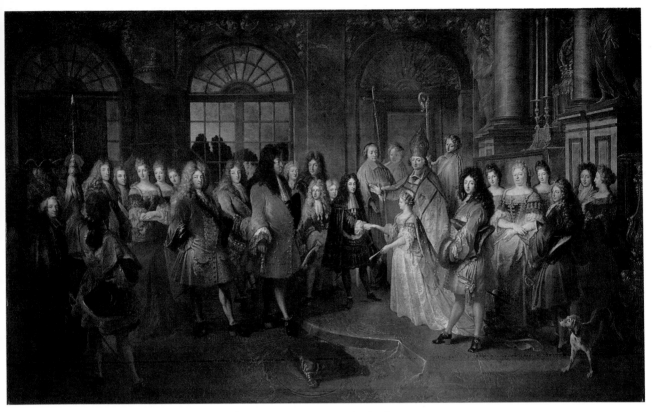

5 Antoine Dieu, 'Marriage of Louis Duc de Bourgogne and Marie Adelaide of Savoy,
7 December 1697'. (Cartoon for the tapestry ordered in 1710).

For the wedding of his grandson to his brother's granddaughter, Louis XIV wore
cloth of gold, as did the bridegroom's father the Dauphin, with his blond wig. The
bride wears the *grand habit* in cloth of silver with a train of royal blue embroidered
with silver lilies. The bridegroom, in respectable black, has an old-fashioned suit
of 1660s style with a doublet and petticoat breeches, retained for weddings as a
now-conservative style. Monsieur is incorrectly depicted, for records show that he
wore a black coat embroidered with gold. Behind him is Madame in a *grand habit*,
the weight of which she complained about, her daughter Elisabeth Charlotte, her
daughter-in-law Françoise Marie Duchesse de Chartres, and her son Philippe Duc
de Chartres. Behind the groom are his brothers Anjou and Berry. The painting
cannot convey the jewels worn at the time. The halberdier in the tabard wears his
hair tied back in the military style which was soon to challenge the periwig. *(Musée
de Versailles, cliché des Musées Nationaux)*

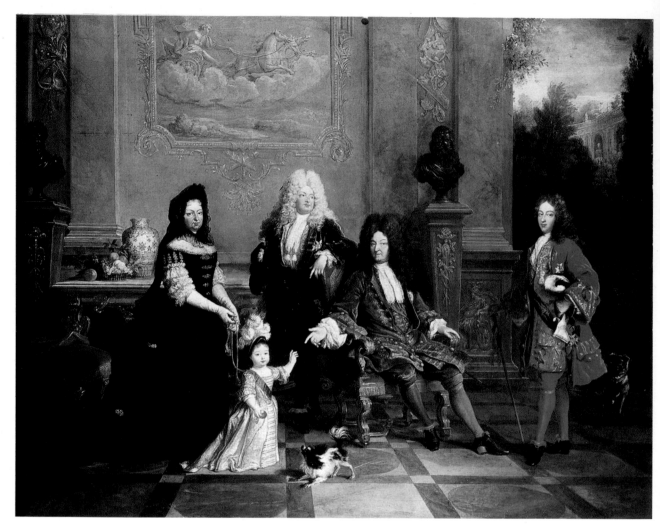

6 Nicolas de Largillière, 'Louis XIV and his Heirs', 1710.
In his old age Louis XIV reverted to the vertical pockets of the 1680s, although
here he is fashionable in matching his waistcoat to his coat cuff. The towering
periwigs worn by Louis and the Dauphin are challenged by the lower wig of Louis's
grandson Louis Duc de Bourgogne, who favours the lower look of the new
generation, and wears low-heeled shoes in contrast to his grandfather's block heels.
He also sports a steinkirk cravat, unlike his elders. The busts represent Henri IV
and Louis XIII. The governess in the black *grand habit*, the Duchesse Ventadour,
was the granddaughter of Louis XIV's governess Madame de Lansac. Her charge
the infant Duc de Bretagne wears ostrich plumes and the ribbon of the order of the
Holy Ghost to indicate his royal status. Ironically, by 1712 all the heirs portrayed
here had been killed by disease, or by their doctors. *(Reproduced by permission of the
Trustees, The Wallace Collection, London)*

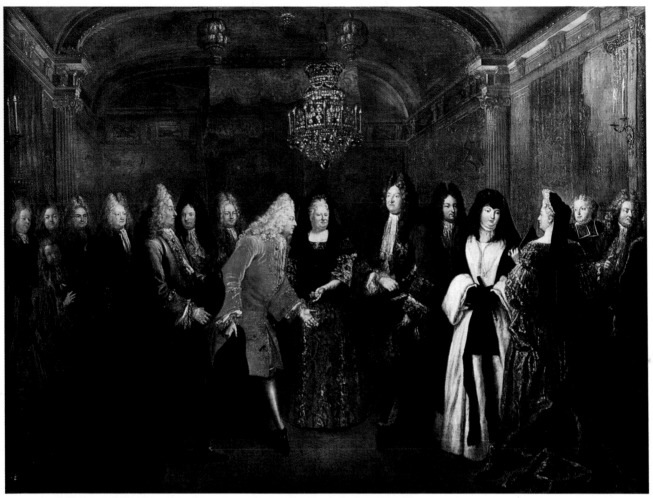

7 Louis de Silvestre, 'Dowager Madame presenting the Elector of Saxony, Frederick
   Augustus, to Louis XIV at Fontainebleau on 27 September 1714'.
   The court comes out of mourning to receive the Elector, but the widowed Duchesse
   de Berry, the Dowager Madame's granddaughter, has to remain in her widow's
   peak and black and white coat. The painting shows the impact of British fashion.
   The lady on the right, in the cloth of gold *grand habit* with silver ruffles, has the
   single-tier cap of British type, while Dowager Madame has a British hoop
   underneath her golden petticoat. Her *grand habit* is black velvet with silver sleeves
   and ruffles. Louis XIV wears the usual brown coat of his later years, with the
   vertical pockets of the 1680s. *(Musée de Versailles, cliché des Musées Nationaux)*

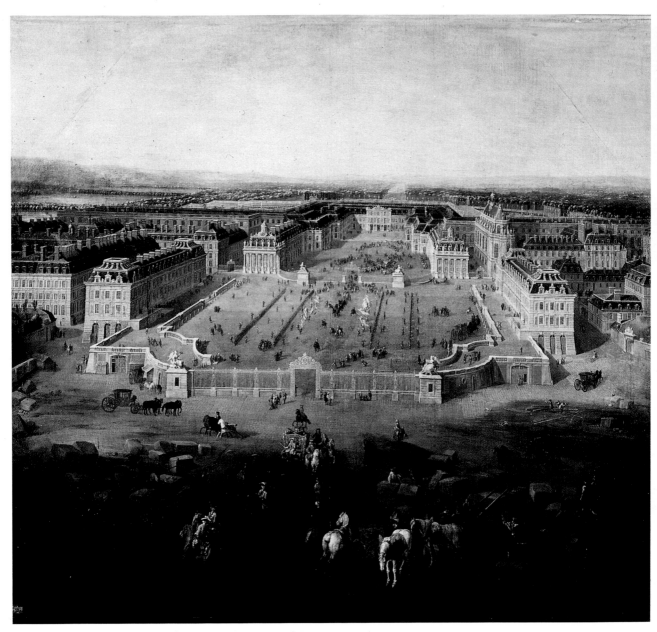

8 Jean Baptiste Martin, 'Versailles', 1722.
   The château de Versailles was completed only at the end of Louis XIV's life, so the
   site was never free of workmen and labourers during his reign there. Firstly Le Vau
   enclosed his father's hunting lodge, then Mansart added the immense wings over
   1678-1708, and the chapel was built last. During the Regency, Versailles was
   abandoned, and Louis XV returned there only in 1722. Louis XIV intended
   Versailles to impress the world, and succeeded, for his fellow monarchs built
   similar palaces in Germany, Austria and Russia. As the temple of the Sun King
   it still attracts visitors. *(Musée de Versailles, cliché des Musées Nationaux)*

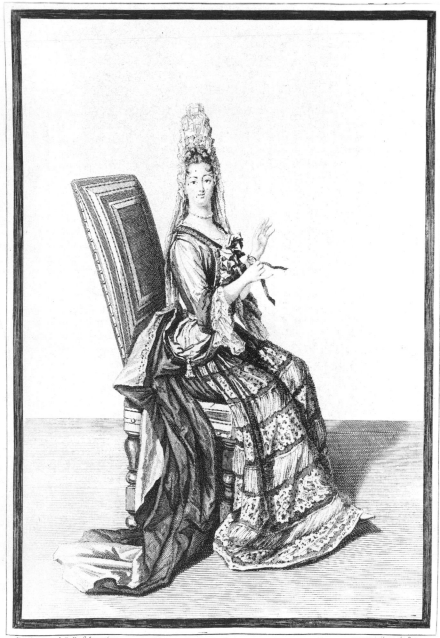

Dessine par I·D·De S·Iean 1693·   *auec priuilege du Roy*

Dame de la plus haute qualité

se vend a Paris sur le Quay Pelletier a la Pomme d'Or au premier appartement

64 Jean de St Jean, 'Dame de la plus haute qualité', 1693. The lady of highest degree wears her commode in four tiers, and the lappets or *barbes* (lit. beards) reach down to her waist at the back. Her manto shows the same contrast lining as the previous illustration, but she has concealed the lacing with ribbons. Her petticoat with stripes of lace and fringe echoes the 1680s and is still being worn in 1696, but a simpler alternative has appeared (above). The importance of the train saw the introduction of a support in the form of *culs de crin*, horse-hair bottoms, which gradually grew bigger to form bustles. (*Victoria and Albert Museum, London*)

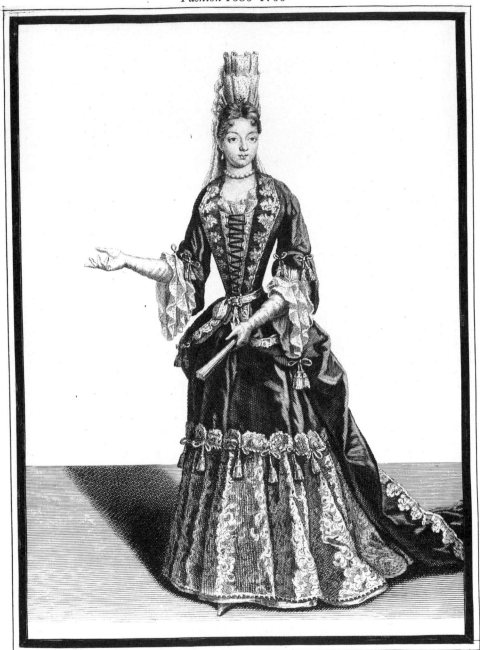

Madame la Duchesse de Bourbon.

se vend à Paris chez A. Trouvain rue St. Jacques au Grand Monarque attenant les Mathurins avec Privil. du Roy.

65 André Trouvain, 'Madame la Duchesse de Bourbon', *c.* 1696.

By the middle of the decade the waist grew a little longer and was tightly laced. The bustle means that trains can be larger and more richly decorated, but the duchesse also must have some hip pads to achieve so wide a hipline. There is no attempt to conceal the front lacing of the manto. Alternating rows on the petticoat are on the way out, and a contrasting panel is employed here, the top scalloped and tied with tassels. The commode has changed from four tiers to two but has not lost height. (*Stadtmuseum, Munich*)

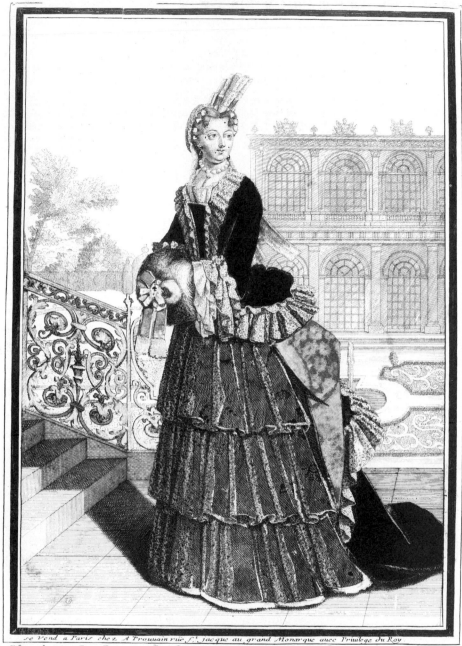

se vend a Paris chez A Trouvain rüe S.t. Jacque au grand Monarque auec Priuilege du Roy.

Charlotte Landgrave de Hesse Cassel Reyne de Dannemarc, fille du Landgrave Guilleaume, et d'Hedwige Sophie Princesse E.le de Brandebourg.

66 André Trouvain, 'Charlotte Landgrave of Hesse Cassel Queen of Denmark', *c.* 1696/7.

The bustle grows more prominent, and trains are built up into a cascade of velvet, silk and lace. Here a dark velvet manto is edged with a gold or silver lace which then sweeps down the train in lively play. The trend for simpler decoration of the petticoat is shown in the net frills with no other elaboration. The commode continues to be in two tiers but has developed a forward lean. Building up the hair into a tower has ceased, and two curls on to the forehead have become the principal style. Lappets or *barbes* remain waist length at the back. (*Victoria and Albert Museum, London*)

Versailles was not even finished when Anne Marie left, for Dangeau noted on 31 May 1685 that there were still 36,000 labourers working on the palace and gardens. Mortality among the labourers ran at about 100 a year. From her mother Marie Adelaide learned of a gigantic court, which required a kitchen, the Grand Commun, housed in a separate building, of 2,000 staff to feed it. Because of the quarter system Primo Visconti said there were 7,000 office holders at the palace, although most of 10,000 guards were accommodated outside in barracks. On ceremonial days 15,000 persons could squeeze into the building which must have made the court seem something like a railway terminus during the rush hour. From little Savoy it looked unbelievable. A peace treaty was trumpeted, Victor Amadeus II quit the League of Augsburg (only to rejoin it later), and the marriage contract was agreed. One of the little girl's bodices was sent to Madame de Maintenon so she could start ordering the bride's wardrobe in France. As the duke was penniless, Louis XIV paid for the dowry, although the duke was happy to run up bills with his subjects for her trousseau which came to 53,905 francs, half of which was for lace and linen, 13,000 for the brocades and 3,000 for embroidered petticoats. Fifteen years later the tradesmen were still petitioning to be paid. This was typical; many an aristocrat refused to pay bills. As a former governess Madame de Maintenon oversaw the establishment of the young princess's household, appointing her own cousin Comtesse de Mailly as dame d'atour (mistress of the robes) along with the Marquis de Dangeau as chevalier d'honneur, the Duchesse de Lude as dame d'honneur, and Comte de Tessé as master of the horse, all for a child of 11. The groom Louis, eldest son of Monseigneur the Dauphin, was 14, so the consummation of the marriage was delayed until 1699 when he was 17 and his wife 14. The wedding was on 7 December 1697, two days after Marie Adelaide's twelfth birthday.[16]

It was the most exciting occasion at court for years, for Madame de Maintenon provided the king with a life of bourgeois domesticity, and the courtiers were very bored. Louis XIV decided that Marie Adelaide would wear the *grand habit* as her bridal gown, in cloth of virgin silver, embroidered with silver, with a train and a coronet of pearls. The weight caused the child to stumble, but Dangeau and Tessé carried the eight-metre train and helped her discreetly. The groom wore a very conservative suit, a good 40 years old in style: a short doublet, and petticoat breeches, which were now sufficiently ancient to be respectable and

formal. It was in black velvet, the usual wedding colour for grooms, embroidered with gold, and had diamond buttons. With it was worn a cape of black velvet, also gold embroidered, lined with cloth of silver. His shirt was white satin. Louis XIV himself gave up his now usual brown for a coat of cloth of gold embroidered around the waist in 'hair colour'. The groom's father Monseigneur the Dauphin wore cloth of gold too. The bride's grandfather Monsieur was in black velvet embroidered completely with gold, and wore his greatest diamonds. The step-grandmother Madame was very annoyed about the weight of her clothes. She was in a cloth of gold *grand habit* patterned with raised flowers in black chenil, and she wore her diamonds and pearls, but found the weight exhausting. There were so many people she had to wait for a quarter of an hour at each door to proceed through the apartments. She was accompanied by her daughter-in-law the Duchesse de Chartres in a *grand habit* of gold brocade, embroidered with silver; her sister, another of Louis XIV's illegitimate daughters, Madame la Duchesse de Bourbon in a *grand habit* of flame velvet embroidered with silver and diamonds; and Louis's daughter by La Vallière, the Princess de Conti in a green velvet *grand habit* embroidered with gold, and bejewelled with diamonds, rubies and pearls. The groom's young brothers the Duc d'Anjou and the Duc de Berry were in gold brocade and in black velvet decorated with golden flowers respectively. Madame loyally wrote to Aunt Sophia with all the details, although what she felt about being escorted by three of the king's bastard daughters surpassed polite expression, and *Le Nouveau Mercure Galant* devoted a massive article to the wedding, to impress the world. Louis XIV ordered the court to look rich, so 5,000,000 francs were spent on silks and jewels. The Duc and Duchesse de Saint Simon Vermondois spent 20,000 livres on their clothes. There was such a demand for dressmakers two duchesses resorted to kidnapping to obtain the women they wanted, so desperate were they to beggar themselves in order to please the king. Louis ordered two court balls to celebrate the union, where the dresses were priced at 12,000 to 30,000 francs each. First, on Tuesday 10 December the new royal duchess had to receive a visit from the exiled Old Pretender aged 11 and his mother, for which she wore a *grand habit* in pink satin embroidered with silver, and a set of diamonds. For the first grand ball the new duchess wore a cloth of gold *grand habit* bedecked with the best diamonds in the crown jewels. The

Dauphin wore a suit of cloth of gold embroidered with silver trimmings. The Duc de Bourgogne wore a black velvet suit, and his brothers Anjou and Berry wore coloured velvets, all three covered with diamonds. Monsieur wore the same black velvet coat and diamonds that he wore to the wedding, an example of royalty being able to get away with wearing the same outfit twice whereas anyone else would have been asked if they had purchased their clothes at a second-hand shop. His son Chartres wore the same sort of golden suit as the Dauphin, and his daughter-in-law and her sister were both in cloth of gold *grand habits* decked with golden buttonholes, and petticoats which the journal called an 'inexpressible richness'. The courtiers were mainly in brocades, or velvets embroidered or appliquéd. At the second ball the Duchesse de Bourgogne wore black velvet covered with diamonds, while her firmament was so full of diamonds and pearls that she dazzled the eyes. Madame wore a *grand habit* of black velvet with a petticoat of gold brocade embroidered with gold. Monsieur was in a suit with silver brandenburgs and buttons of rubies and diamonds. Chartres wore a black velvet suit which also had brandenburgs down the front in gold and diamonds, lined with pink velvet, with the sleeves covered with silver lace. The Dauphin and his sons were in gold brocades.

The young duchesse was allowed to enjoy herself to the full. On 18 August 1698 she and her party went off in four coaches with eight horses each, to Paris to visit the Fair at St Denis. She wore a linen-grey manto decorated with frills, and decked with silver lace, emeralds and diamonds. Two large diamond pendants on her forehead were matched by her earrings and necklace. She visited Asanville who sold ribbons and jewels, Le Maire who sold porcelain and La Frenaye who sold gold knick-knacks. She then watched the rope dancers and marionettes, and her step-uncle Chartres escorted her home.[17] The linen grey of her manto represents the brief fashion for off-white at the end of the 1690s. Chartres wore a coat of grey-white at the wedding.

Madame, since the defeat over her son's bridal choice, was not going to see her daughter Elisabeth Charlotte sacrificed to one of Louis XIV's bastard sons, and had pressurized the king and Monsieur into selecting a proper prince. In 1698 she won; Leopold Duke of Lorraine was accepted as spouse for young Elisabeth Charlotte. A proxy ceremony took place at Versailles first. Monsieur as father of the bride wore a suit of cloth of gold with silver buttonholes and trimmings, with black satin ribbons with diamond tips at the shoulder and sleeves. The bride's mother Madame was described by the reporter as 'noble et modeste' and that was all. The Duchesse de Bourgogne attended in a *grand habit* of silver tissue in flame and green, and wore her diamonds. For the ceremony of introduction the bride was escorted by the Marquis de Blainville, grand master of the ceremonies and M. des Granges, master of ceremonies. She wore black Tours silk embroidered with gold, and a petticoat of cloth of silver embroidered with gold and a hint of flame. Her train was 6½ ells long in gold Spanish point lace, and she wore a diamond necklace and firmament tower. The Duke of Lorraine was represented by the Duc d'Elbeuf who wore the same historical suit as Bourgogne had done, namely a doublet and petticoat breeches in cloth of gold decorated with purple flowers, the cloak lined with purple and trimmed with silver lace. Next day came the contract ceremony. Elisabeth Charlotte wore virgin white in the form of a *grand habit* in cloth of silver, which was trimmed with silver lace, as was the petticoat. Her parure was of diamonds and rubies. The proxy groom Elbeuf had a doublet and petticoat breeches of black velvet patterned with golden flowers, and appliquéd with gold Spanish point lace. The petticoat breeches were decked with three fills of the same lace, and gold and blue ribbons, in the style of 1660. The Duchesse de Bourgogne attended in a *grand habit* of linen-grey damask embroidered with silver flowers, and decorated with diamonds and emeralds.

The bride's trousseau was displayed in Monsieur's gallery according to French custom, after Monsieur had fussed everything and everybody into order. There were 15 dresses in assorted brocades, 7 embroidered dresses, 15 embroidered petticoats and 12 underskirts. One dress was of black velvet with a border of golden garlands over a foot deep, with a petticoat of cloth of silver embroidered with two kinds of gold. The weight was considerable. The linen was all trimmed with Venetian point lace, and embroidered with the cipher of the Duke and Duchess of Lorraine. Louis XIV gave a *grande parure* of diamonds, that is a complete set with tiara, earrings, necklace, pectorals and bracelets. Monsieur gave three parures, one of diamonds, one of rubies and diamonds, and one of other stones. The king also gave a set of gold brocade furnishings, and Monsieur a *toilette* dressing table with mirror in gilded vermilion by M. de Launay.

On 16 October 1698 the bride Elisabeth Charlotte paid a tearful farewell to Madame Elisabeth Charlotte her mother, her father Monsieur, and her brother Philippe Duc de Chartres. Duke Leopold of Lorraine set off from the opposite direction, and the couple met at Vitry on 23 October. For this occasion the duke wore a blue suit decked with gold galloons over a finger wide, a gold brocade waistcoat and red stockings. The couple proceeded to his capital Nancy for the official entry, when Elisabeth Charlotte the younger wore her heavy gown and found it so incapacitating that she was obliged to change afterwards because she could not stand up in the dress. The amount of decoration on court clothes was becoming self-defeating. Madame had complained about it for years but found if she refused to wear gold-embroidered velvets, the tailors embroidered the underskirts and made them just as heavy. Sophia of Hanover had already expressed her sympathy for the late queen Marie Thérèse in 1679 when she saw the weight of embroidered bullion the poor consort had to wear. Baroque ornamentation was becoming too ornate and ponderous and a reaction was going to take place. The first signs could be seen in the lightweight Chinese style of ornamentation which the court designer Jean Berain began to introduce around this date. In the meantime princesses and duchesses had to stagger beneath the weight of ceremonial grandeur, while the men's golden suits were not much lighter.[18] Louis XIV was going to insist that such finery be worn right up to the end of his reign, but even he was to find it all too much to carry. Understandably the style of the regency of Philippe Duc de Chartres was to aim for lightness and informality after 1715. But no one could foresee that in 1698. The succession looked secure. The king had his son the Dauphin, who had three sons. Everyone now looked to the young Duchesse de Bourgogne to do her royal duty and produce an heir in the fourth generation but her dancing at balls until dawn only encouraged miscarriages. Louis XIV was not concerned. He had plenty of heirs.

Madame's German relations used her as their fashion information bureau. In December 1691 she had to reply to a request from her cousin's husband Frederick William, Elector of Brandenburg, who wanted a pattern for a hat aigrette. Madame replied that the elector was wrongly informed. Nobody at Versailles was wearing aigrettes in the hat. She had seen only one example on an Opéra dancer. What men wore in the hat were diamond buckles to hold the feather, and large diamond clasps to hold up the brim. Four years later Madame wrote to say that hairstyles were still high but not quite so high as before, and the commodes were now inclining in front, so that a leaning tower replaced the vertical one. In October 1699 the *Gazette d'Amsterdam* reported that the little Duchesse de Bourgogne had tried to please Louis XIV by devising a lower commode without any lace pinners, or *barbes*, literally beards, hanging down to the neck, when it was customary to have four such pendants. The Princesse de Conti happened to enter the room soon afterwards in an ordinary commode, and comparing the two, Louis XIV preferred the lower kind. Accordingly, the court took them up for a while, and the new commodes were termed the *petites Bourgognes*. It was, however, only a temporary adjustment. Even larger commodes were to blossom after 1700, and the king's dislike made no great impact. Moreover, lacemakers had a vested interest in keeping laced caps in vogue. The adoption of the *petite Bourgogne* at court was so instant, that a week later when a few ladies arrived in the former commode wishing to see the king dine, they looked so different that they appeared to be creatures from another world, and withdrew in dismay. It meant that seamstresses had to work over night when all the ladies at court wanted to change their headdresses at the same time.[19]

Louis XIV pulled rank when it came to taking the little Duchesse de Bourgogne for afternoon outings, when she had finished her school lessons. Poor Monsieur her grandfather was excluded from their drives. All along the king had said that the bride of his grandson was his special concern, seeing in the vivacious youngster something of her grandmother Henriette Anne for whom he had felt such a strong attachment. What the child herself felt about her over-scented, high-heeled grandfather, she was too polite to say. Her presence at court did cheer things up, and Louis XIV was now ordering masked balls, dances, outings, plays, all to entertain his great-niece, and granddaughter by marriage, Marie Adelaide. Even her father-in-law the Dauphin did not see as much of her as the king, or her teenage husband Louis Duc de Bourgogne who still had sessions with his tutors. The duchesse herself knew from her mother that the person she had to please, amuse, divert most at Versailles was the king.

FIVE

Conclusion 1700–1715

Louis XIV could flatter himself that his fashions had reached as far as Russia. When Czar Peter the Great returned to Moscow in 1698 after his visit to the West, he ordered his male subjects, with the exception of priests and peasants, to cut off their beards, give up their long coats, and to dress in the western manner. To the top of Russian society this meant in the French style, as can be seen by the Muscovite embassy to Turkey in 1701, but the British ambassador recorded that they were still uncertain about how to wear it:

The Muscovite Ambassador and his retinue have appeared here so different from what they always formerly wore that ye Turks cannot tell what to make of them. They are all coutred in French habits, with an abundance of gold and silver lace, long perruques, and, which the Turks most wonder at, without beards. Last Sunday, bcing mass in Adrianople, ye Ambassadore and all his company did not only keep all their hats off during ye whole ceremony, but at ye elevation, himself and all of them pulled off their wigs. It was much taken notice of and thought an unusual act of devotion.[1]

There was more to looking French than clothes. One should read all the new volumes on etiquette, which said that periwigs should be worn at all times before one's superiors, when only the hat should be removed. Hats should also be doffed before the portrait of a social superior, and when receiving a letter or messenger from the king. And of course one had to stand in the presence of royalty, which at Versailles meant most of the day for the courtiers. Only duchesses had a right to stools, the *tabourets*. The exception was for the select few invited to Marly-le-Roi where the etiquette was informal.

The reckless spending at court continued, as if France had not been at war for almost 40 years. Maréchal Vauban pleaded for a fairer taxation system, which did not put most of the weight of Louis XIV's wars and magnificence upon the poor peasantry. For this honest concern, he was dismissed from court,

despite a lifetime of devoted service. No criticism was allowed. The lavish expenditure now centred upon the young Duchesse de Bourgogne at 14. The New Year and century saw a masked ball for her at Marly-le-Roi where she appeared as Flora, covered with silk flowers, with her nymphs, whom Madame thought the costume suited less well. The Dowager Princesse de Conti led a group dressed as Amazons. The Duchesse de Chartres led a troup of sultanas attired in oriental splendour. Another party represented Spaniards in black velvet, with quantities of diamonds. Next day there was another masked ball at which the Duchesse de Bourgogne did not dress up but wore her *grand habit*. The theme was the Savoyards, with people dressed as villagers, but perhaps the young duchesse fclt that it was below her dignity to appear as one of her father's subjects. There was also a balletic interlude with Harlequin, Ponchinella and Marinetta.

On 27 January, Louis XIV gave a masked ball at Versailles. The Duchesse de Bourgogne changed her costumes three times, coming firstly as Flora again, then as a milkmaid, and lastly as an old crone. The king retired at 2 a.m. but she stayed up dancing until 4 a.m., which was typical. On 4 February she led an entry at Marly-le-Roi dressed as a Spaniard in black velvet, probably with some collar or ruff to hint at the golilla. A humorous entry followed with the Duc de Chartres and the Princesse de Conti as an old schoolmaster and his wife, with four children, played by adults, and four nannies. Next day at another masquerade the Duchesse de Bourgogne appeared as a magician, in robes covered with plants, stars and moons. The centrepiece of this evening was a masquerade about Don Quixote and his adventures. The young duchesse asked the chancellor to give her a ball, so the Comte de Pontchartrain obliged with a comedy, then a collation served in an unusual arrangement of stalls like a market, with courtiers dressed as a French patissier, a Provençal orange and

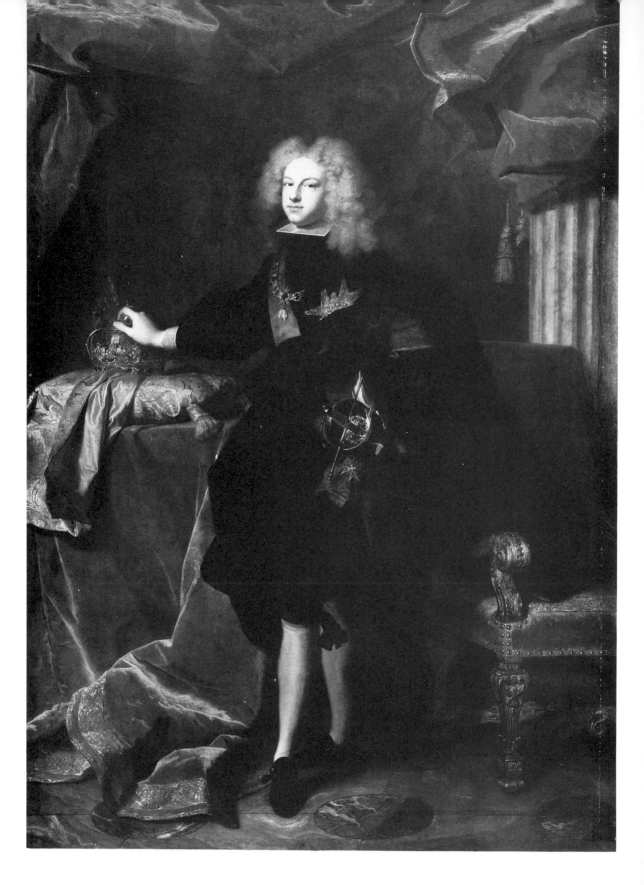

lemon merchant, an Italian lemonade seller, a French sweetmaker, and an Armenian coffee, tea and chocolate man. A grand ball followed until 4 a.m.

On 13 February M. le Prince gave the duchesse a ball at Versailles, when she appeared as a masked sultana, doubtless veiled and decked with diamonds. The buffet here was a spectacular Chinese fantasy designed by Jean Berain, who was responsible for everything from carrousels to state funerals. A comic foursome, including the king's bastard son the Comte de Toulouse, arrived in taffeta farthingales, with identical wax masks, and turbans, so it was impossible to detect which was which. 17 February saw a masquerade devised by the Duc de Chartres, this time for Monseigneur the Dauphin, which represented the Grand Signior with his menagerie. The Marquis d'Antin was carried on a palaquin like the sultan, surrounded by slaves and sultanas, who included Monseigneur's daughter-in-law. Soon after this a Venetian masquerade was mounted, where everyone had to dress as characters from the *Commedia dell'arte*. And so it went on, every season, night after night: incredible expenditure on costumes in cloth of gold and silver, embroidered, with bullion or jewels, quantities of costly lace, miles of brocade and silk never mind the fringes, frills, appliqué work, sequins, spangles, and ostrich plumes; all to ensure the most exposed parade of wealth, to make other courts feel shabby, to prevent the aristocracy from having any money left for other activities, and to flatter Louis XIV.[2]

In December 1700 the courier arrived from Madrid. Carlos II had died and bequeathed all his empire to one of Louis XIV's grandsons, on the advice of the Pope. Louis XIV had already signed an agreement with William III to divide the Spanish possessions with Austria in order to prevent war, but Louis XIV now broke it. He accepted the will of Carlos II, and chose his second grandson Philippe Duc d'Anjou as Philip V of Spain. A portrait of this

French king in full Spanish court dress was ordered at once from Rigaud, but it was an empty gesture. Philip V was going to ban the black Spanish court suit and golilla. Louis XIV in fact advised Madrid that Philip V should wear Spanish dress, but his grandson had other ideas. After all he had been raised amidst the magnificence of Versailles, and anything so old fashioned and sober as Spanish court dress was not to be tolerated. Within three months of his arrival Philip V had banned it except for magistrates and officials who continued wearing golillas into the early nineteenth century. The French were hoping to make huge profits out of a new fashion for French clothes and fabrics, and to end the large British sale of baize to the Spanish. With the French king went the *grand habit* for ladies, and it was goodbye to plain hairstyles. Spanish grandees who refused to adopt French dress were deprived of their privileges. The struggle between the two types of costume had lasted for a century, and now in 1700 French luxury emerged victorious over Spanish sobriety. But it all meant another war. William III was furious that Louis XIV had broken their attempt to find a peaceful settlement, and the Austrians were not going to allow all their American possessions to pass to the French without a fight, so they invaded Spain. In 1701 William III organized the Grand Alliance against France's expansion into Spain. The War of the Spanish Succession was to occupy most of the remainder of Louis XIV's reign.

As if to escape from this horrendous prospect, fashion developed a passion for frills, and fluffy innocence now came to the fore. The furbelow or falbala frill decked petticoats in three or four rows; it ran down the revers of mantos, it adorned the cuffs, and tumbled down the edge of trains. In sympathetic style bed canopies, chair seats, curtains all sprouted frills to match those on capes and commodes. Frills were even attached to the *cul de crin* or bustle, with a particularly obvious standing frill which gave the effect of a duck's tail sticking up; this made a significant difference between the silhouette of the 1690s and that of 1700. These furbelows could be in any fabric, such as patterned silks, satins, or else in lace and embroidered stuffs.

The frill even spread to commodes, and the *barbe* returned despite the Duchesse de Bourgogne's attempt to extinguish it in 1698. It gained in importance when a frilly pendant down the side of the face became a dominant feature, and this style of commode was dubbed a *rayon* because it was like the

---

67 Hyacinthe Rigaud, 'Philip V of Spain in Spanish Court Dress', 1700.
A cynical gesture by Louis XIV's second grandson Philippe Duc d'Anjou to whom Carlos II bequeathed his crown. Although he is portrayed in sober Spanish court dress with the golilla collar he abolished them when he reached the Spanish court. Thereafter only the magistracy had to wear them. At the court it was French luxury conquering Spanish pride (see fig 8) and a French dynasty on the throne, but Philip would have to fight to retain it. (*Louvre, Paris; cliché des Musées Nationaux*)

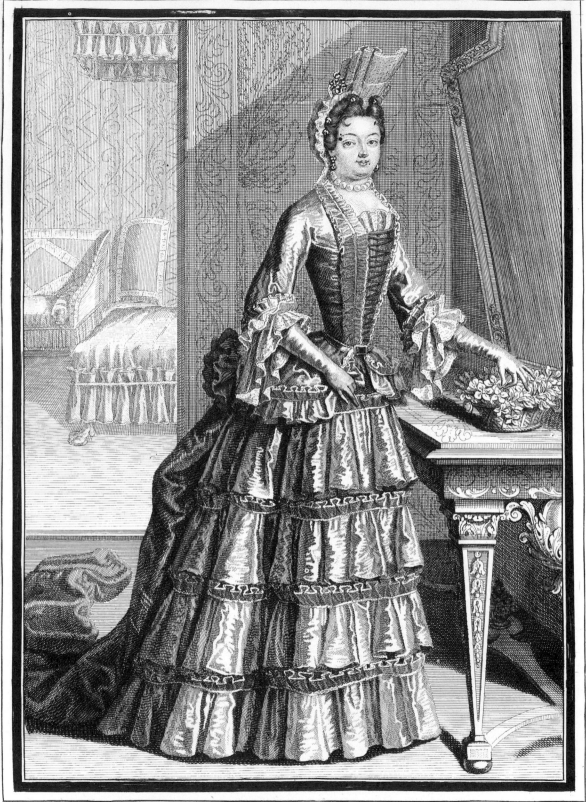

Madame l'Electrice de Brandebourg.

A Paris chez J. Mariette rüe S.ᵗ Jacques aux Colonnes d'Hercules avec Privil. du Roy.

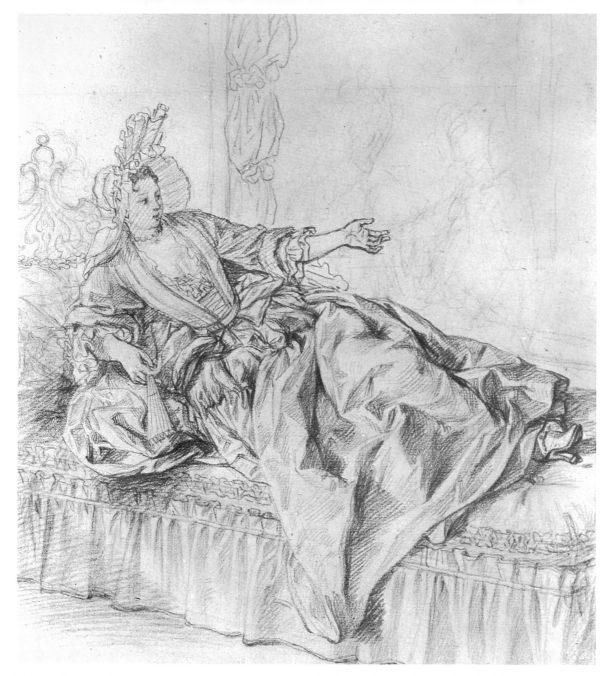

68 J. Mariette, Madame the Electress of Brandenburg',
c. 1700.
Madame Elisabeth Charlotte's cousin, Sophia Charlotte,
who became Queen of Prussia in 1701. The vogue for
falbalas from 1693 reaches its extreme in 1700 when there
are four rows of frills on the petticoat, a frill of ruching down
the revers of the manto, and more frills down over the
bustle. The bedchamber furniture in the background has
also donned frills in sympathy. The very tight lacing of the
bodice can be seen in the strain on the silk. Patterns are out
of favour and plain fabrics dominate. The commode
continues its forward lean but refuses to grow smaller.
(*Stadtmuseum, Munich*)

69 Bernard Picart, 'A Lady Resting', 1703.
The development of the *rayon* version of the commode with
the frill at the edge of a cap expanded out like rays of the sun,
hence its name. Far from disappearing, as Louis XIV
wished, commodes were worn even larger. The manto too
was now 40 years in fashion, but showed no sign of fading
away regardless of the king's dislike. The overall look has
become simpler with no patterned fabrics, and frills have
been reduced to a tuck in the petticoat at hip level.
(*Reproduced by Gracious Permission of Her Majesty The Queen*)

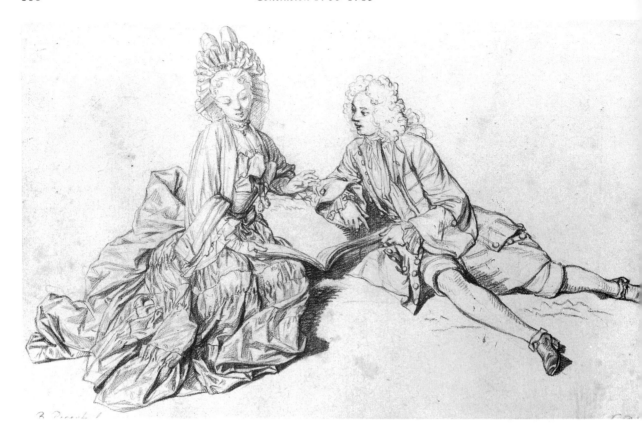

rays of the sun. Height was beginning to yield to width, so the towering construction of lace and wire shrank, as the face frill grew. The ears were concealed now and the hair was no longer piled up in front with artificial *tours*. By 1708 the *rayon* was the most common form of headdress to wear with *habit de ville*. While the king's dislike of commodes was well known, the *rayon* could claim to honour King Sun's symbol.

In February 1702 the Duchesse de Bourgogne Marie Adelaide received a Spanish costume from her sister Marie Louise, named of course after her murdered aunt, who at 12 had been selected as bride for the embattled King Philip V of Spain. Madame Elisabeth Charlotte, the girls' step-grandmother, approved of the Spanish costume and said it suited Marie Adelaide. It was decently covered, for a start, for the shoulders were draped with satin and the neckline was square. The narrow sleeves ended in lace frills as was usual, though the number was greater than in France; silver lace was mixed with Venetian point lace so that it resembled the wide flounces actors and actresses wore on stage. The bodice laced down the back, which Madame considered the proper way,

70 Bernard Picart, 'Figures for a Galanterie', 1708.
The frills of the rayon have become more formalized and the tiers behind it have been reduced to one; the trend is to leave the face more clear. Plain fabrics continue modish for both sexes, and the only decoration on the petticoat is two rows of standing frills. Women's sleeves grow wider to match the pagoda sleeve on men's suits. The back silhouette now has a duck's tail effect as the train is fixed to stick up over the bustle. The young man has tied his wig back in the military way. His knee rolls can clearly be seen. (*Ashmolean Museum, Oxford*)

71 J. Mariette, 'Marie Thérèse de Bourbon Princesse de Conty'.
The new silhouette with the duck's tail effect achieved by standing frills on a cape, over the stiffening of the bustle. Frills abound on the petticoat, for there is both an apron with three tiers of frills and a petticoat with three tiers of fringed frills. Summer saw a vogue for muffs of peacock feathers. The amount of frills suggests a date closer to 1700, but this plate has been located next to the previous one to show the silhouette after 1700. (*Stadtmuseum, Munich*)

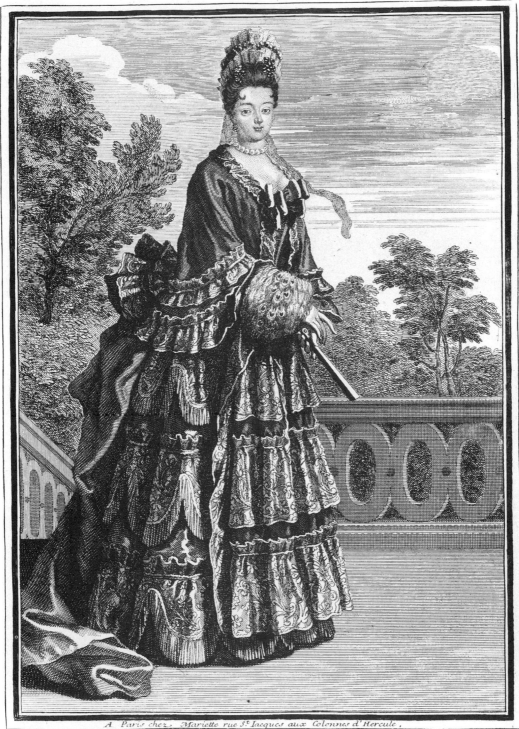

A Paris chez, Mariette rue St Iacques aux Colonnes d'Hercule.

Marie Therese de Bourbon Princesse de Conty

Fille d'Henry Iules de Bourbon, Prince de Condé et d'Anne Comtesse Palatine est née le jer février 1666. a épouse François Loüis de Bourbon Prince de Conty le 29 juin 1688.

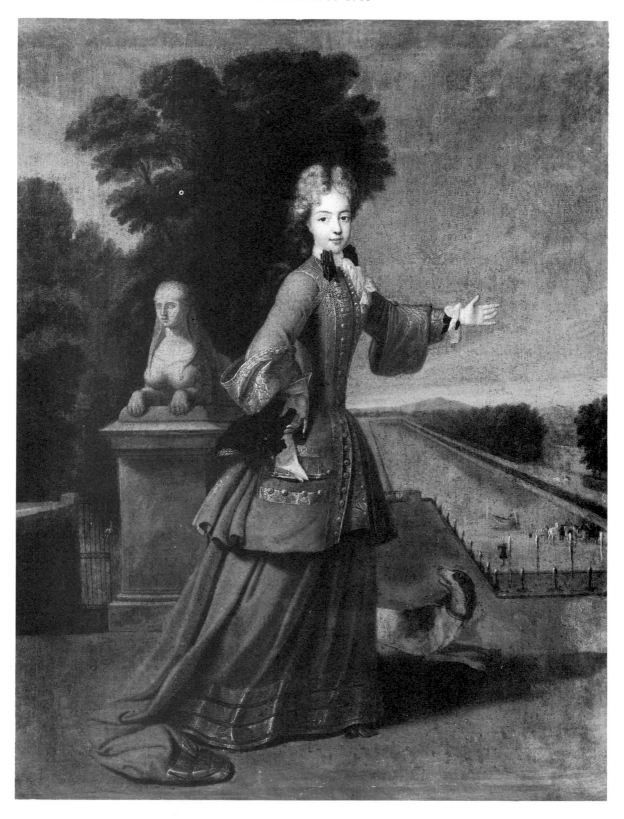

like stays rather than front-lacing mantos. The underskirt was still formed of iron hoops in the persistent Spanish way although much narrower than farthingales had been. Wide at the hem and narrow at the waist, these hoops produced a more triangular effect. The costume was in cherry-coloured satin covered with silver lace. Madame wondered if it would spark a new fashion, but it did not yet do so.[3] The country which revived wide-paniered skirts was not Spain or France, but Britain. It was enough to give Louis XIV a seizure, but it was a clear indication of who was winning the war. The more the Duke of Marlborough trounced Louis XIV's invincible army, the more famous Britannia became, and the more influential her fashions.

It was in January 1709 that Isaac Bickerstaff in *The Tatler* denounced these new 'giant petticoats' that could not get through doors, and were as large as canopies of state. He could see no sense in the fashion although obviously whalebone merchants, rope-makers, weavers, fabric warehouses would all do well out of the extra material and support involved. As the Press commented on hoops in January 1709, they must have come out in 1708, and were distinct from the Spanish model by being wide at the hips. Despite the hostilities, hoops *à la Britannique* crossed the Channel and appeared at Versailles. The Duc de Saint Simon was astounded. These immense rotundities, as he called them, were unbearable. What had possessed French youth that it should wait with such impatience for British madness to be imported to knock them silly? Louis XIV was even more horrified – British hoops at court, when Britannia was leading the Grand Alliance against him! Madame was most amused. She wrote: 'He could never forgive the French ladies for affecting English fashion!'[4] She was now 57 and did not take to paniers herself, except in a modified way, but it pleased her British ancestry considerably to see the silly French, as she called

them, falling for the fashion of their major enemy. The huge impact of hoops changed the silhouette completely, and this is why they caused such a sensation. Height and baroque towers were tumbling before a wider manifestation. The change in emphasis was well illustrated by an anonymous panegyric describing the alteration, issued in Bath in 1711; *The Farthingale Reviv'd: or, More Work for the Cooper*:

> Oh Garment, heavenly wide! thy spacious Round
> Does my astonish'd Thoughts almost confound!
> I own, the Female World is much estrang'd
> From what it was, and Top and Bottom chang'd:
> The Head was once their darling constant Care,
> But Women's Heads can't heavy Burdens bear,
> As much I mean, as they can do elsewhere.
> So, wisely they transfer'd the Mode of Dress,
> And furnish'd t'other End with the Excess.[5]

A horizontal look was coming into vogue and the late Baroque stress on grand verticality was being undermined. The tall person like the king had had a good run since periwigs, and high heels for men had appeared in 1661, but now Louis XIV was ageing, and the desire began to emerge for a less dominating figure. While Louis XIV wore his red high heels until he died, the younger generation changed over to a lower look from around 1709–10 and a shorter stature came into fashion as the new century sought a new image for itself. Obviously, if the Baroque had been grand, vast, heavy and high, then the new period could look different only by being informal, smaller in scale, less opulent, and more lightweight and playful in style, a development which is now termed Rococo art.

The change was gradual. Periwigs attained their greatest dimensions after 1700, flowing down almost to the elbow, and rising to two peaks over the forehead. The alteration came from the army which was forced to tame periwigs, for no officer could afford to have his vision blocked by a periwig blowing across his face when the enemy were charging at him full pelt. As early as 1697 the military were tying their periwigs back off the face into a bow at the neck. By 1706 when Marlborough routed Maréchal Villeroi at Ramillies, both the English and the French cavalry were wearing bag wigs, with the wig ends caught into a black silk bag at the neck. Both sides found the bag wig very practical during conflict. Consequently the first bag wigs to appear at Versailles were worn by officers reporting from the front. Louis XIV did not adopt them. Civilians appearing before him still had to wear periwigs like the king, but the military were

---

72 P. Gobert, 'Marie Adelaide of Savoy Duchesse de Bourgogne', *c.* 1707.
After being the star of the court in her teens, Marie Adelaide grew tired of all the dressing up involved, and the constant changing, so she started to copy her step-grandmother Madame by wearing her hunting habit for day, and the *grand habit* for evenings. The hunting livery was scarlet with a golden braid trimming. The simple jacket and skirt combination was much easier to operate in than the heavy, ornate clothes of ceremonial occasions and festivities. To those who had to endure it, Louis XIV's luxury could begin to pall. (*Versailles, cliché des Musées Nationaux*)

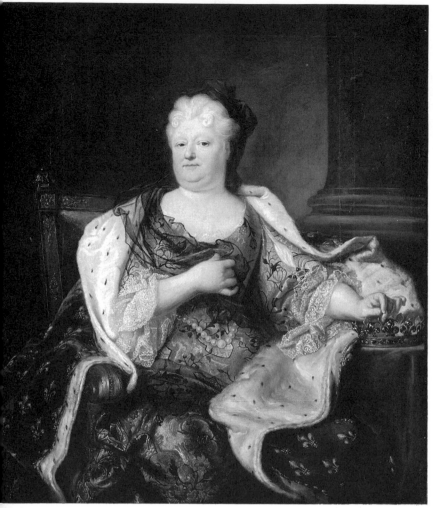

73 Hyacinthe Rigaud, 'Madame Elisabeth Charlotte Dowager Duchesse d'Orléans'. Madame was delighted with the news that Queen Anne had reduced commode caps to one tier, and was very amused when Versailles copied them. A critic of extremes in dress, Madame's own white hair is now very much in the fashion. Her costume displays artistic looseness but in reality she was a firm believer in stays and lacing. Her letters about events at Versailles are invaluable. (*Versailles, cliché des Musée Nationaux*)

sporting an alternative. It was only a matter of time, waiting for the king to die, before bag wigs could be worn at court, but the young outside, wishing to identify themselves by looking different, took to the bag wigs very quickly, although there were social restrictions on where and when they might be worn. The periwig continued to be worn for ceremonial occasions right down to the French Revolution, although in a shorter, tighter-curled version, for the Age of Reason liked order, and the Baroque taste for tumbling curls looked too wild. The bob wig became the tamed descendant of grandiose periwigs.

The new institution of the three-piece suit rode on in triumph unassailed. There was no composition of clothes to replace it. As women had bustles, and from 1708 hoops, the rear of the coat had to undergo some expansion to keep up with the change of emphasis, and to meet the new definition of fashionable shape.

Accordingly the number of pleats in the coat skirts was increased, with more pleats inserted at the sides, and they were reinforced with stiff lining to give a fuller line. Coat tails could now swing as a man turned, so he could give a dramatic twist akin to that made by bustled ladies, albeit in an abbreviated garment without a train. The fullness of a man's skirts was to

74 Nicolas de Largillière, 'Philippe Duc d'Orléans with a Portrait of Madame de Parabère', 1703.
Madame's imperfect son, the former Duc de Chartres, who succeeded to his father's dukedom in 1701. The casual style of the future Regent was going to have a big impact on court fashion, for he strongly disliked the formalities of Versailles and much preferred Paris. Louis XIV would never have been portrayed with an open shirt and his cravat undone. Philippe's white-powdered wig is tied back in the military manner which was to make periwigs redundant outside the court. (*Toledo Museum of Art, Ohio*)

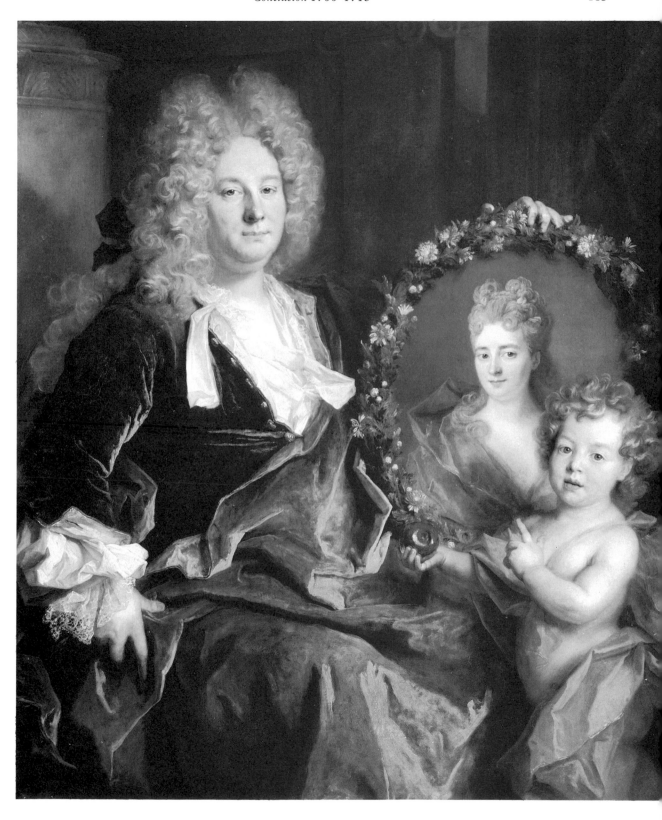

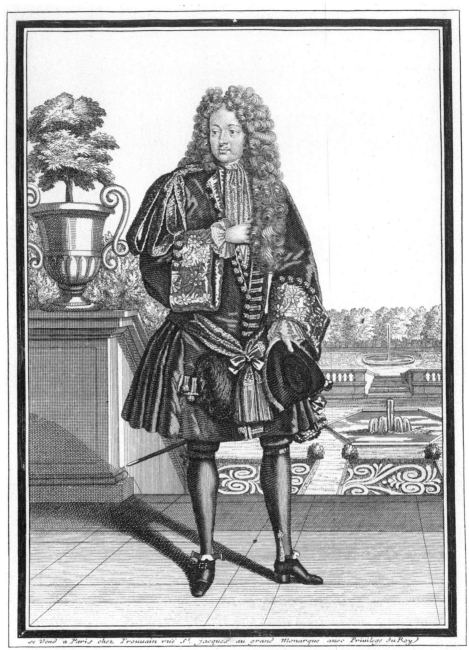

se Vend a Paris chez Trouvain ruë St. jacques au grand Monarque avec Priuilege du Roy)

Frideric III Electeur de Brandebourg
Duc de Prusse de Magdebourg de Cleve de Pomeranie &c.

75 André Trouvain, 'Frederick III Elector Brandenburg, Duke of Prussia', *c.* 1700.

The husband of Madame's cousin who became King of Prussia in 1701. His coat is plain apart from the cuffs of floral brocade which had a short vogue around 1700. The number of pleats in the coat skirt reflect the bustles worn by women, for the fashion for back interest affected both sexes. Clocked stockings and knee rolls continue, and pockets have settled down to the standard flap like a marshall's portfolio. Hats are becoming smaller, and shoe heels are less high. A lower look is creeping in. (*Stadtmuseum, Munich*)

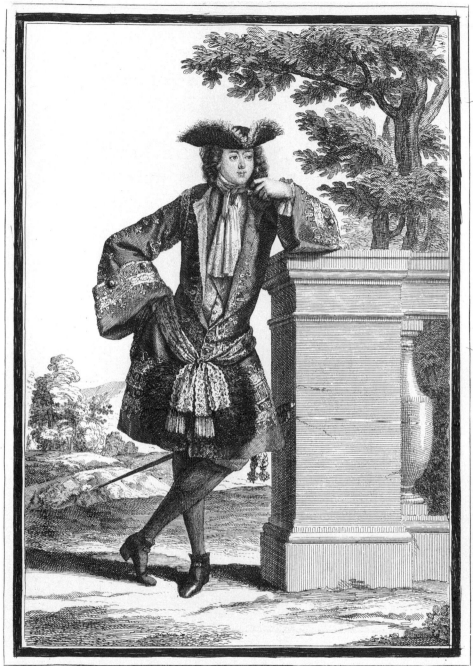

Loüis Auguste de Bourbon Duc du Mayne.

A Paris chez J. Mariette rue St Jacques aux Colonnes d'Hercules avec Priv. du Roy.

76 J. Mariette, 'Louis Auguste de Bourbon Duc du Mayne', *c.* 1705.
Louis XIV's favourite bastard son Maine, whom he tried to give a large role in the future regency. He wears an embroidered suit with the pagoda sleeves still in vogue. Enormous muffs remain fashionable from the 1690s. His hat is the mathematical cock with three equal sides in a triangle termed the tricorne. His loose cravat shows the younger generation's yearning for some informality and his wig is tied right back. (*Stadtmuseum, Munich*)

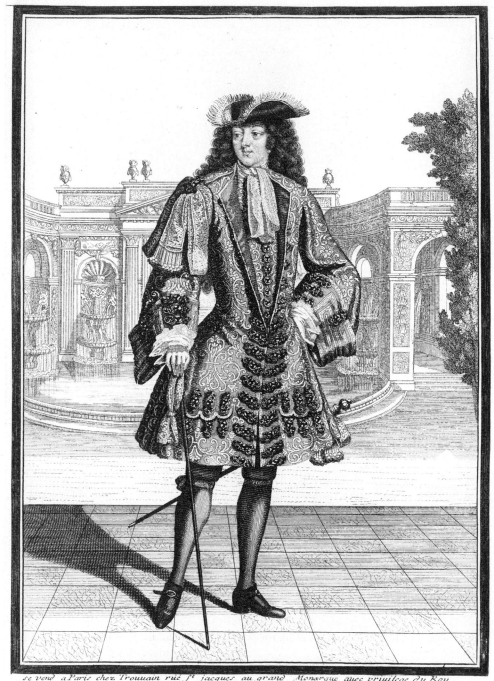

se vend a Paris chez Trouuain rüe S.t Jacques au grand Monarque auec priuilège du Roy

Monsieur le Duc de Bourbon[73]

77 André Trouvain, 'Monsieur le Duc de Bourbon'.
The diamond clasps down the coat, on the cuffs and pocket flaps, and the diamond buttons down the vest, show the richness still required at court where wealth had to be displayed. The heavy silk distinguished the wearer from the masses in woollen cloth. The width of men's coats begins to echo the new hoops for women. Stockings and knee rolls must be worn tight without a wrinkle. (*Stadtmuseum, Munich*)

continue even further, for once hoops widened the figure, men began to widen by the insertion of wires into their coat tails, which reached its apogee after the death of Louis XIV, who would probably have banned the development had he lived to see it.

The British favoured their suits plain, so in London unadorned velvet and quality cloth dominated the upper classes, and finery was worn only for royal birthdays. The decorated suit was French, and at Versailles embroidered coats were everyday wear, with the decoration down the front, and around the waist. Where the two countries agreed was on the ornamentation of the waistcoat or vest, although the degree was less extreme in England. Brocade waistcoats were very fashionable in the early 1700s in such combinations as a dark blue velvet suit with a gold brocade waistcoat, a grey velvet suit with a silver waistcoat, or a crimson velvet suit with a waistcoat of gold and silver. The French liked to add sequins, spangles, gold lace, raised embroidery, and of course jewels for parties and ceremonies. Whereas the sleeves of waistcoats and coats had been harmonized in length around 1691, a new disharmony developed after 1700 for the waistcoat sleeve began to grow again until it protruded below the coat sleeve cuff, so that it had to be turned back over it. This resulted by 1710 in a fashion for a brocade waistcoat cuff to cover the sleeve cuff. This was the principal distinction in wearing the coat for about five years, after which the coat cuff was covered with the material of the waistcoat, and the waistcoat sleeve retreated back into the sleeve of the coat. It was a variation on the suit, by matching the waistcoat with the cuff of the coat to show a new colour combination. Louis XIV allowed this fashion at Versailles for he wore it himself, and so did his grandson the Duc de Bourgogne in his presence. As Louis had a waistcoat decorated with braid, braid now appeared on his coat cuff to match; at 72 in 1710, this was one of the new developments which he did adopt, for it did not impose any major alterations on the suit, which he had been wearing for a good 30 years.

Fashion likes to take a modification and turn it into a style. In the middle of the 1680s some men began to turn the bottom of the kneebreeches inside out, to show the lining. The 1690s took this further by pulling the stocking up over the turned-back kneebreeches, instead of putting them and the garter under the kneebreeches. Thus knee rolls were born, and after 1700 they were padded to give them a rounder shape. The stockings had to be pulled extremely tight, then the roll smoothed into shape, and the garter fastened very firmly, to ensure a perfect result. It was the typical elaboration of a detail, which working men had no time in the morning to mess about with, but which the aristocratic courtier had a valet to achieve for him. One physical asset which all European males had needed in the West since the Middle Ages was a good pair of legs, and particularly a good calf, for they all exposed their lower limbs. Skinny males could purchase padded stockings if their assets were shrunken, but it was a very sensitive subject, for sometimes the padding could slip. It was a matter about which ladies loved to comment, as was typified by Madame's cousin Sophia Charlotte Electress of Brandenburg and Queen of Prussia. At Luisburg she teased the Italian Count Montalban that the excellent calves displayed inside his hose were not his own. Next day the count burst into her bedchamber and stuck his bare legs on her dressing table to prove that his assets were absolutely genuine. A Latin would bristle at the suggestion that his physical charms were not real.[6]

As the king was ageing the idea of white-haired periwigs began to gain ground. Scented wigs were not new, and they had been perfumed when they first appeared in the 1650s, and different-coloured powders had been used on them too, in red, black, blond or brown. It was only towards the late 1690s that white- or grey-powdered wigs appeared, although Louis XIV never wore them himself, preferring a black periwig to the end of his days. Yet around him white-powdered wigs, and subsequently white-haired wigs, became more common, as if honouring the king's advancing years by making all the court elderly about their heads. There was as always an overlapping period with coloured periwigs and white ones co-existing, but the white-haired wig gradually began to oust coloured ones from about 1715. It was to impose a uniformity of head colour upon society which endured down to the 1760s. Everyone who could afford wigs had to have them in white or grey, which shows the standardization of society, and the tendency away from displays of individuality which characterized the Age of Reason. In contrast, Louis XIV had lived through a period of wild abandon, with the wigs in any colour. The Baroque period shared something of the character of the Romantic movement which was to rebel against the uniformity of the eighteenth century, for it had allowed for personal expression and some excess.

It was essential for Britain to have a Protestant

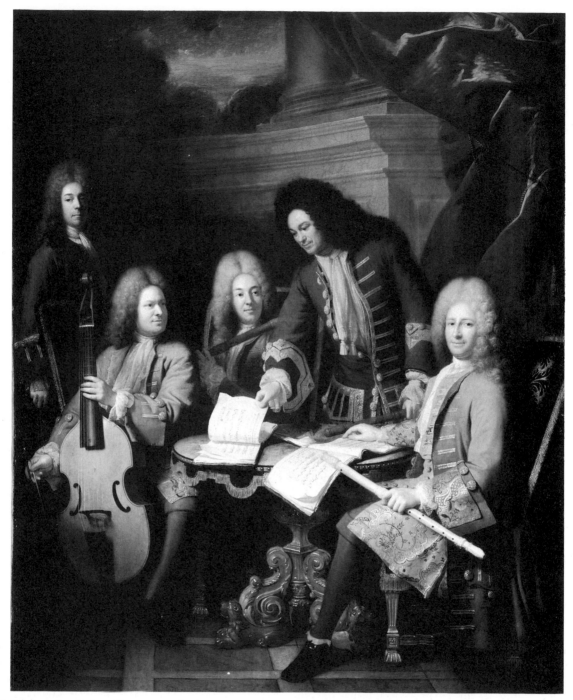

78 Attributed to Robert Tournières, 'La Barre and Other Musicians', *c.* 1710.

The group sits around the music of La Barre's trio sonatas of 1707. It suggests that La Barre was a liveried servant to the rich amateur on the right. Outside court, cloth suits dominate, but the amateur wears the newest variation where the vest sleeve again grows longer than the coat sleeve, and has to be turned back over the cuff. This style dominated the last five years of Louis XIV's reign, and led eventually to cuffs being covered with the fabric of the vest. It was to be the last fashion Louis XIV wore. Periwigs are being tamed and shortened as the new century prefers neatness to grandeur. Shoes are becoming flat after 50 years of block heels. (*National Gallery, London*) succession if she was to defeat Louis XIV's plans to put a Catholic on her throne, but in 1700 William III's nephew William Duke of Gloucester died at 11. He was the only one of Princess Anne's 14 children to reach that age. William III had had no children by Mary II, and now it did not look as if her sister could produce living children. The heir to William III was Princess Anne herself, but after her? The Catholic line of the Stuarts had been exiled, so William had to look for the Protestant Stuarts. Back in 1613 James I and VI had married his daughter Princess Elizabeth to Frederick V, Elector Palatine and head of the Union of Protestant Princes which had been founded by his father Frederick IV. This marriage produced 13 children of whom six died in childhood. Of the seven who survived only two had reached the eighteenth century: the nun Louise Hollandine, Abbess of Maubuisson, aged 78, and her youngest sister Sophia of Hanover, aged 70. The direct legal line of male Palatines had died out following the deaths of their brother Charles Louis in 1680 and of his son Charles without issue in 1685. Of their other brothers Prince Maurice had been lost at sea, Prince Rupert of the Rhine had a daughter, and Prince Edward had left two daughters. William III, however, was looking for soldiers to continue the fight against Louis XIV, and the only one of the Palatines with sons was Sophia of Hanover who had six: George Louis, Frederick August, Maximilian, Charles Philip, Christian and Ernst August. William III went to meet Sophia at Het Loo and in 1701 published the Act of Succession naming Sophia and her sons as heirs to the British throne. Sophia was now a widow dressed only in black, for her husband Ernst August had died in 1698: George Louis was now the Elector of Hanover. Sophia was also a grandmother, for George Louis had been married to his cousin Sophia Dorothea, and their son George August was born in 1683. He was now 17 and grandmother was looking about for his bride, whom she arranged in 1705 to be Caroline of Ansbach. Their son Frederick, the future Prince of Wales, was born in 1707. Thus Sophia could offer the British throne three generations of heirs: George I, George II, and Frederick, father of George III, and they were all Protestants. William III died in 1702 and was succeeded by Queen Anne, whom Sophia and George Louis visited in 1705 when George was created Duke of Cambridge. Sophia was also the mother to Prussia through her daughter Sophia Charlotte and was to arrange a marriage between George Louis's daughter Sophia Dorothea and

Sophia Charlotte's son William Frederick Crown Prince of Prussia. Thus the Palatines were making a comeback. If Louis XIV had occupied their homelands, they had found two other thrones, through Sophia, who was called the wisest women in Europe by her librarian von Leibnitz, no less. There was also a link to the Orange House of the Netherlands, for Sophia's grandmother had been Louisa Juliana of Orange, daughter of William the Silent, and great aunt to William III, and this link was to be renewed later in the century by the marriage in 1734 of George II's daughter Princess Ann to another William of Orange.

All such dynastic arrangements were gall to Louis XIV, but if he could make schemes so could other people. As his mother had said, he never thought about other people's feelings, and seemed annoyed that countries which he invaded should dare to object. Yet it was his attacks which forced bigger states to come into being. Sophia's husband the Elector Ernst August did not divide his lands among his eldest sons in the German tradition but introduced the right of primogeniture, so that Hanover was born as a united state. Louis XIV had not expected that, nor did he foresee that Prussia would expand from Brandenburg, but he brought such changes about by invading Germany.

There was gloom at Versailles in the last years of Louis XIV's reign. In 1701 Monsieur died of a stroke after a gigantic row with his brother over Louis's broken promises. Louis had pledged that if Monsieur's son Philippe married his illegitimate daughter he would award him all sorts of privileges, but it had not happened, and Madame could snort that it served him right for ever agreeing to Louis XIV's scheme. Louis had broken promises to Philip IV, William III and his brother. The death of Monsieur meant that his son Philippe became Monsieur the Duc d'Orléans and his wife Madame. His mother Elizabeth Charlotte became the Dowager Madame and dowager duchess. She had been wearing mostly black already as a mature lady of 49, but was obliged to don full French court mourning, with a linen band across her forehead to conceal her hair, a white coif on top, and pinners. A long linen veil fell into a train seven ells long. Her dress was a black mourning coat with wide sleeves, which had white ermine down the front and around the cuffs, and a broad band of ermine at the hem, with an ermine train seven ells in length. All her women were put into long mourning coats of black crépe, and Dowager

Madame wrote to Aunt Sophia in Hanover that they were a ghastly sight.[7] Etiquette required a royal widow to take to her bed to receive visitors; mirrors and pictures were removed, black hangings replaced tapestries, and black crêpe over the windows produced a gloomy light. A widow could not attend plays for two years and had to remain indoors as a recluse but Elisabeth Charlotte was able to occupy herself with all her weekly letters to her daughter in Lorraine, to her step-daughter in Savoy, and to Aunt Sophia and all her German cousins. She did not approve of the freedom that Louis XIV and Madame de Maintenon were allowing the Duchesse de Bourgogne with so many late night parties. The duchesse bore a son at last in 1704, but he died the following year of convulsions, and Elisabeth Charlotte thought his mother's lack of discipline a contributory factor. She herself received happier news from Lorraine, of a grandson Louis who survived for five years. She would have been even happier, but she did not live to see the event, over the marriage of her grandson Franz of Lorraine, born 1708, to Empress Maria Theresia of Austria, and his election as Holy Roman Emperor. There were 13 Lorraine grandchildren but most died of childhood diseases.

Le Nouveau Mercure Galant became increasingly sad reading, with long lists of aristocratic mortalities at the front, beside which the regular paeans of praise for Louis XIV's wisdom, honesty, fortitude and honour, seemed particularly inappropriate, although they were compulsory, since it was he who was sending so many Frenchmen to their deaths. The court was kept greatly in ignorance, defeats were not mentioned and information was restricted, so it could take months for people to build up a true picture of the disasters the French Army was now suffering. The courtier could watch the couriers galloping up covered in mud, and could see the king looking serious, without knowing where the battle had been, who won, and the effect. The Dowager Madame found it most frustrating. The luxurious propaganda was required to continue regardless. She moaned that she had to attend the Carnival in February 1706, when her mourning was over, being expected to dress up in fancy clothes at her time of life, as she was entering her 54th year. She disguised herself under a huge length of green taffeta attached from a long stick, to make her seem tall and slim, whereas she was by now decidedly stout. Louis XIV could not tell who it was, and grew annoyed at being saluted by someone he could not identify. The young, of course, still enjoyed dressing up, so the Duc

de Bourgogne with three others disguised themselves to look like ornate lampstands in gold with silver sashes and gold masks, with candelabra on top of their heads, and stationed themselves at the four corners of the room. The Dowager Madame did find that quite witty. The Dauphin was also amusing by wearing a woman's cap with pinners hanging down the sides of his face.[8]

Further masked balls were required to celebrate the birth of a second son to the Duc and Duchesse de Bourgogne on 8 January 1707, Louis Duc de Bretagne. He survived immediate infancy, so hopes were high for his eventual succession to the throne. It was not to be. Marie Adelaide's sister Marie Louise Queen of Spain produced a son in 1707, Louis Philip Prince of the Asturias, so more balls were ordered to celebrate the event.[9] Louis XIV could congratulate himself on two great-grandsons, the heirs to two thrones, even if war was waging to deprive them of those destinations. 1708 was also the worst winter of his reign. Europe shivered under a devastating frost that killed cattle, crops, vines and people. At Versailles fur-lined coats and ermine petticoats became fashionable at once. France was on her knees and Louis XIV sued for peace, but the British government insisted Philip V must leave Spain. Louis XIV would not agree to that, so the war resumed. Even the French were calling Marlborough the Invincible. Lille, which Louis XIV had himself captured back in 1668, fell to the Allies; the greatest fortress Louis had created surrendered to Marlborough. Other fortresses followed.

Disasters on the battlefield were soon matched by disasters in the dynasty. In 1711 the Dauphin, Monseigneur, succumbed to smallpox. The palaces were in chaos, but even so the Dowager Madame, Saint Simon recorded, 'dressed again, in her *grand*

---

79 Alexis Simon Belle, 'Matthew Prior', *c.* 1716.
The diplomat Prior was secretary on the diplomatic visits of Lords Portland and Jersey to Louis XIV, and in 1711 Queen Anne appointed him Plenipotentiary Minister in France. His coat shows the impact of the embroidery pattern of the *justaucorps à brevet* upon diplomatic dress. While Prior has none of his sleeves, the embroidery on his coat skirts and pocket flaps is entirely in the justaucorps tradition which affected such coats into this century. He is allowed a fashionable touch in the turned-back vest sleeves over the cuffs, but periwigs have to be full in the old pattern, not in the tied-back versions now worn outside court. The letter to the King indicates that Prior wore the coat at court. Lace instead of fringes now edges gloves, but knee rolls have become an institution. (*St John's College, Cambridge*)

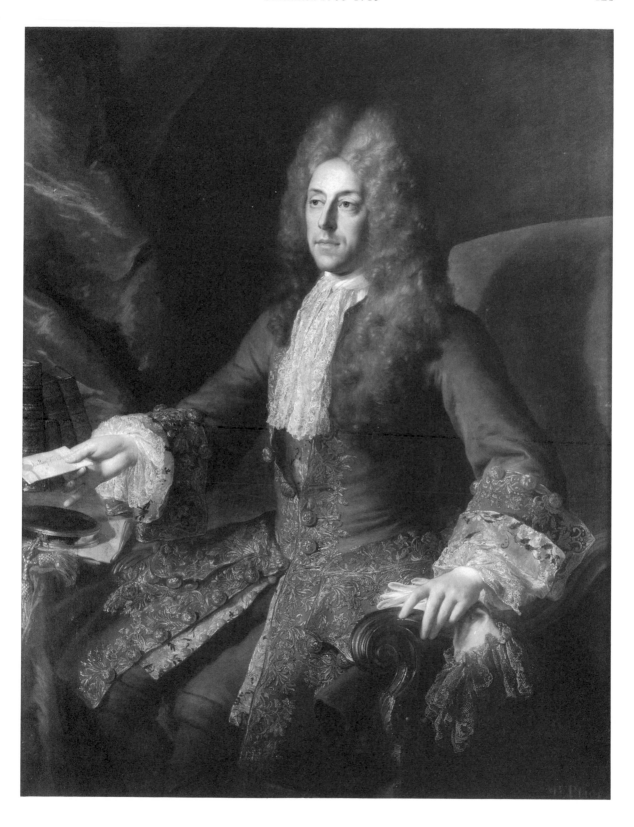

habit, and arrived howling . . . furnishing the bizarre spectacle of a princess who redons full ceremonial costume in the middle of the night, to come and weep and mourn amidst a crowd of women in nocturnal undress, almost in masquerade.'[10] The Dowager Madame was always correctly dressed for the occasion. Funerals could spark off squabbles. Long mourning cloaks were required for royal funerals, but when the Prince de Conti died in 1709 his family told the dukes to wear long mourning cloaks, which they refused to do, and turned up in only mourning suits. The only mourners in long cloaks were the Conti themselves, trying to claim the rights of a first prince of the blood.

There was now a new Dauphin and Dauphine, the Duc and Duchesse de Bourgogne, who fortunately had another son, baby Anjou, in 1710. Marie Adelaide began to sober up as she neared 26. She had grown tired of all the dressing up of her youth, and began to copy her step-grandmother the Dowager Madame by wearing hunting habits during the day and the grand habit in the evening and for receptions, with undress in her apartments. The king and Madame de Maintenon did not approve, but the treasurer Desmaretz told them that Maintenon's cousin the Comtesse de Mailly was mostly responsible, for she was lazy, extravagant and incompetent, and had run Marie Adelaide's wardrobe very badly; she was dismissed. Madame Quentin, wife of Louis XIV's barber and perruquier, took over.

The amount of splendour still worn in Paris and at Versailles astounded foreign visitors. Marlbrough had broken through the Ne Plus Ultra lines in the north and the Austrians had occupied Madrid but at court: 'Every body dresses with a World of Finery. *Ribbands, Lace*, and *Looking-Glasses* are three things without which the French cannot live. Gold and Silver is become so common, as I've said before, that they shine upon the Habits of all Degrees of Persons, and immoderate Luxury has confounded the Master with the Servant.' The ladies certainly need not worry about burglars,

because they carry their whole Fortune upon their Backs. The Quality Trail behind 'em a long Tail of Gold or Silk, with which they sweep the Churches and the Gardens. All of 'em have the privilege of going maskt at all times, concealing or shewing themselves when they please. With a Black Velvet Visor they go sometimes to Church or to a Ball or Play, unknown to *God* and their *Husbands.*

The wearing of masks to protect the complexion from the sun went back to the sixteenth century.

It was no different in Paris at the Jardins des Tuileries, from which common folk were excluded. 'The Ladies in Fashions *ever new*, with their Adjustments, their Ribbons, their Jewels, and agreeable manner of dressing, in stuffs of Gold and Silver declare the continual Application of their Magnificence. The Men, for their Part, as vain as the Women, with their *Feathers* and their *Fair Wigs*.'[11] The anonymous reporter even accused the French of such levity that they invented new modes of dressing every day. He was writing about changes of detail, the position of a bow, the length of a plume, the size of jewellery, the number of patches worn on the face. The principal trend did not alter, with hooped skirts gradually growing wider, and men's coat tails spreading out in sympathy.

Versailles was still glamorous enough for Sophia of Hanover in 1706 to have ordered bridal clothes for her granddaughter from Paris, despite the war, and despite the fact that her sons and grandsons fought against the French on the battlefield. Her neice the Dowager Madame was asked to order the trousseau as she would know all about the best *grand habits*, mantos, commodes, accessories, and suits for the males. Elisabeth Charlotte also sent an ivory face-scraper for removing excess powder, which Sophia thought would be most useful in Prussia where everyone wore too much powder, and kissing was too common, so that an embrace could result in suffocation. Sophia would dearly have liked to attend the wedding in Berlin, but at 76 could not face the winter journey, so there was a proxy wedding first in Hanover for grandmother, with George August representing Crown Prince Frederick William, and a second wedding in Berlin in November when Sophia Dorothea espoused the Crown Prince. She caught a cold, so was excused from wearing the bare-shouldered *grand habit*, and the king allowed her to appear in the manto at the celebrations, which were clearly designed to impress Versailles.[12] Thus the Germans were attracted by the magnificence of the French court, and longed to equal it, even while they detested Louis XIV and his policies. King Sun suffered a severe blow in 1712. Firstly his grandson the Duc de Berry went down with measles, but recovered. By 5 February Marie Adelaide the Dauphine had it. She was bled and given emetics, which of course made things worse, and she died. The Dauphin Louis soon showed signs of the infections, and was given the same treatment. He died. Both their sons caught the infection, Louis Duc de Bretagne now five, and Anjou aged two. The doctors set to work on the elder, and by their bleeding, purges and emetics finished him off by 8 March. The children's governess Charlotte Eleonore Madeleine de la Motte Houdancourt, Duchesse de Ventadour, who had been recommended by Dowager Madame for whom she had been a maid of honour for 16 years, locked the doors and would not allow the doctors to bleed the baby Duc d'Anjou. He caught the fever but he survived, thanks to her. There would be a Louis XV.

The king and the court were too stunned to react. Three direct heirs had been wiped out in one year. The epidemic also claimed many lives in the palace and in Paris. Madame de Maintenon said God had unleashed the disease to teach Louis XIV humility. Others accused the Duc d'Orléans, Philippe, of being ambitious for the throne and killing off his relations, which Louis XIV and Dowager Madame both knew was vicious nonsense. Dowager Madame knew her son was not perfect, for Philippe was pleasure-loving, easy going, too fond of drink and women (thus the total opposite to his father) but absolutely incapable of murder. All the courts of Europe were astounded by the developments, and much rethinking had to be begun. If Louis XIV was reduced to one heir in his great grandson generation would his second grandson Philip V be summoned to the French throne if that baby should die? The Allies own case underwent an embarassing alteration. The smallpox that killed Monseigneur also killed the Emperor in Vienna, which meant that the Allies' candidate for the Spanish throne, the Archduke Charles, then occupying Barcelona, had to dash back to Austria to become Charles VI, leaving the Alliance without an immediate candidate. Britain and the Netherlands did not want to see one Hapsburg ruling Austria, Germany, Hungary, Spain and the Americas, any more than they wanted to see one Bourbon ruling France, Spain and the Americas. New negotiations had to be started. Ambassadors were despatched. In 1713 the Duke of Shrewsbury arrived in Paris with his wife. Saint Simon declared that the duchess was fat, masculine, and a faded beauty who still thought she was attractive. She spoke loudly in bad French, and her manners were silly, yet her magnificence and general familiarity made her the fashionable star. Within weeks she was able to do what Louis XIV had been unable to effect in 28 years.

Although Queen Anne had worn the tall commode when young, by about 1710 she and her ladies at the British court introduced a much lower headdress with the tiers reduced to one. This was much safer, for the tall commodes often caught fire from candles. In 1703 the old Marquise de Charlus was gambling with the Archbishop of Paris Le Tellier and the Prince de Conti, and as she leant forward over the table her commode touched the candles and started to flame. The Archbishop quickly knocked the headdress off, but unfortunately dislodged the old lady's wig at the same time, which horrified her as much as the accident. Similarly in November 1707 the Dowager Madame, after a hard day's hunting, fell asleep at her writing table, and her commode caught fire from the candles on the table as her head nodded forward. She awoke to find burning sparks raining down on her scalp and eyebrows, but her yells soon brought her ladies to her aid. Such accidents were only too common, and doubtless some periwigs caught fire the same way, so the lower headdress of the British court was a safety measure of some value.[13]

The Duchess of Shrewsbury took this lower headdress to the French court. She told the French ladies that the headdress at Versailles were too big and ridiculous, and they listened. Saint Simon was amazed and so was Louis XIV. The commode

was a construction of brass wire, ribbons, hair, and of all sorts of trinkets, more than two feet high, which put women's faces in the middle of their bodies, and old women wore them the same, but in black gauze. Whenever they moved the aedifice trembled, and the inconvenience was extreme. The King, so much a master even down to the tiniest things, could not stand them; they lasted for more than ten years [actually 28] without his being able to change them, no matter what he said or did to bring about their extinction. What this monarch could not do, the taste and example of a silly old foreigner executed with the most surprising rapidity. From the extremes of height, women threw themselves into the extremes of flatness, and headdress which are much simpler, and more convenient, and sit much better on the head, endure up to today.[14]

The low cap succeeded so spectacularly because it expressed the change from Baroque verticality to the horizontal ideals of the new century. Louis XIV received another lesson that female fashion was not his slave, and that the ladies would change only when that change was in keeping with the general alteration in mainstream style. The absolute monarch was not so omnipotent as he thought, and a British headdress, and British armies, showed it. The power of the latter reinforced the effect of the former, so that British hoops, British headdresses, and British suits were a reflection of British authority. Saint Simon might feel a personal insult that foreigners were daring to set the style, when France was the centre of the universe, but it was an expression of political fact.

Wits could make much fun out of the word *commode*, for as well as the headdress it also meant commodious, so one could joke about the incommodity of commodes. Saint Simon approved of the low caps because the were 'plus commodes' than commodes had been. For the sake of simplicity I have kept to one name for the construction, but it was also known as the *freland*, the *frelange*, the *tour*, and lastly the *rayon*. The first two names referred to the bonnet and pinners being worn together. *Flandan* was a kind of pinners joining with the bonnet. For the last two years of Louis XIV's reign the low caps he had long demanded were worn, but as Dowager Madame remarked he never forgave Frenchwomen for adopting British styles, despite the fact that he himself had been wearing a British-type suit with the coat and vest to the knee and narrow kneebreeches, for a good 30 years. He had probably found it convenient to forget the origins of the suit in 1666, but now British commodes were proving an unwelcome reminder that not every innovation in dress was born at Versailles.

Of the five granddaughters and one grandson whom Philippe Duc d'Orléans sired, one Dowager Madame found singularly impertinent and lazy: Marie Louise Elisabeth, a drunkard at 15. Yet she was selected as the bride for Louis XIV's third grandson Charles Duc de Berry. Her grandmother lectured her about her gluttony in vain. Because of the war foreign brides were not available for the usual Catholic sources, Savoy and Austria, were fighting against France, and Spain had no daughters. The unsuitable marriage took place in 1710, but following the deaths of the Duc and Duchesse de Bourgogne in 1712, the Berrys were the first couple after the king. There was no queen, the Dauphin little Louis was a toddler, so the Duchesse de Berry was required to be first lady at receptions. She told her grandmother to shove her from behind to make sure that she took up the right position. Even so the Dowager Madame found much to criticize in her granddaughter's appearance, for she turned up in the *grand habit*, with 14 pins of the finest diamonds in the world, and 12 patches on her face. Grandmother informed her that the dress was right, but she had overdone the beauty spots. The first lady in the land should not be covered with *mouches* like an actress.[15] The vogue for patches on the face went back to the 1640s, but continued well into the eighteenth

century. Worries about the Duchesse de Berry's suitability ended in 1714, when the husband, who had survived the measles, died after a riding accident; the widow had to don court mourning and retire from most court events. The court would come out of mourning for important visitors, such as the Doge of Genoa who came to Versailles in 1685 when the court was in mourning for Louis XIV's cousin King Charles II, and now in 1714 for the visit of the Elector of Saxony. The person bereaved, however, like the widow or widower, had to remain in full mourning. Consequently the only surviving grandson was now the second, Philip V, who was attempting to sit on the Spanish throne.

The Allies were most insistent that if Philip stayed in Spain, he must agree to the complete separation of the French and Spanish kingdoms, and return all Spanish territory in Europe, outside Spain, to the Austrian Hapsburgs. The peace treaties took from 1712 to 1714 to finalize. Louis XIV won half a victory in that Philip could have Spain, but he failed to break the remaining Hapsburg ring for Austria took over the Spanish Netherlands and the north Italian duchies, and the German states were stronger than before. He had to recognize the Protestant succession in Britain. Britain also took Newfoundland, the key to Canada, Gibraltar and Minorca where her navy could monitor France and Spain. Luckily for Louis XIV the Allies had not wanted to occupy France, but to push her back behind her borders.

The Duc de Saint Simon was most critical of the clothing of the king's ministers. At the start of the reign clerical black was the proper dress for royal servants of state. As late as 1701 the king's secretary Rose still wore a little cloak, a black satin skull cap, a small collar like an abbé, with the personal habit of sticking his handkerchief between his coat and vest, saying that it was nearer his nose there than in a pocket. Yet Louis XIV allowed his ministers to regard themselves as extensions of himself, so they stopped dressing like servants: 'From there, the secretaries of state and the ministers successively quit cloaks, then the collar, then the black suit, then the plain, the simple, the modest, and finally dressed themselves like gentlemen of quality.'[16] This is certainly born out by the portraits where ministers are as periwigged and cravated as nobles. Colbert had worn mostly black, but made sure his daughters married dukes, so they were nobody's servant. One servant not so affected was the king's personal valet François Quentin, who had quite a family at Versailles. Although he had spent his life among the greatest seigneurs he never adopted courtly manners and graces; a big man, rustic in type, brusque but good natured, he made a perfect valet. His distinguishing mark was that he still kept his moustache whereas Louis XIV had shaved his off about the time of his marriage to Maintenon, and so was one of the few individuals at Versailles who dared not to copy the king. Otherwise moustaches were found only in the army. Dowager Madame thought the moustaches on the king's regiment most becoming when he took her to inspect them on 26 June 1715, as they all had new uniforms in light grey

---

80 François de Troy, 'Louis XIV Receiving the Ambassador of Persia', 1715.
The last occasion, 19 February 1715, when Louis XIV made a ceremonial appearance in the Galérie des Glaces, Versailles. His diamond-covered coat, valued at 12,500,000 livres (francs) was so heavy it made him stoop. His luxurious principle had become a burden in physical fact, quite apart from its economic effects. By the kings's knee is his great-grandson Louis the Dauphin, aged five. In September the little boy became Louis XV, under the care of the Regent Philippe Duc d'Orléans on the far right. The person in black is probably a translator. The Persians under Mohamet Riza Berg wear caftans and turbans. King Sun was now setting. (*Musée des Beaux Arts, Saintes*)

with gold silk frogging and flame-coloured epaulettes. Obviously some flame was still in evidence, given the king's old preference for it, even at the end of his reign.

The scene was changing. In June 1714 the Electress Sophia of Hanover collapsed and died in her garden at Herrenhausen. Her stays were cut but it was too late; she was 84. The family had known its losses, for her daughter the Queen of Prussia had died in 1705, and three of her sons were killed fighting against the Turks. George Louis wrote to Queen Anne that he was broken-hearted at losing such a wise mother, but only six weeks after her death Queen Anne died at 57, and George Louis was proclaimed His Britannic Majesty King George I, in addition to being the Elector of Hanover. Louis XIV had failed to prevent it.

Louis made one last attempt to outshine the sun in 1715, when he received an embassy from Persia. He donned a coat of black and gold embroidered with the finest diamonds in the crown jewels, worth 12,500,000 livres, which was so heavy it forced him to stop. He had to stagger to the throne and gave his illegitimate sons Maine and Toulouse pearls, diamonds and coloured stones so that they too might shine at his side. The opposition to the bastards was

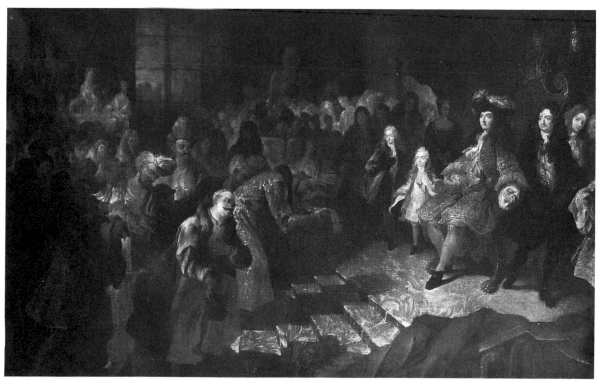

represented by Dowager Madame in a *grand habit*, and her son Philippe Duc d'Orléans in a suit of blue velvet embroidered with a mosaic pattern, overlaid with diamonds, which Saint Simon, a supporter, considered 'a triumph of magnificence and good taste'. Hitherto the king had worn the blue sash of the Ordre du Saint Esprit under his coat for formal occasions, but on this occasion he wore it on the outside, which made every other male present who was wearing the order itch to get away to effect that change himself. The weight of the diamond coat was significant for it made the king seem smaller and by May he was noticeably beginning to shrink. Resplendent clothes which were too heavy to move in had reached their limit.

The scurry began. Louis XIV had already legitimized his bastards to give them a place in the inheritance. Madame de Maintenon pressurized him to appoint Maine as governor of the little Dauphin's education, for she had brought up the illegitimate children, and was trying to block the legitimate candidate for the regency that would be necessary, Philippe Duc d'Orléans. By the end of August 1715 it was diagnosed that Louis XIV had gangrene. His body had begun to decay, although his mind remained lively. Louis XIV knew his nephew would have to be Regent, but he spent more time with his bastard sons. The Duchesse de Ventadour brought little Louis the Dauphin, the future Louis XV, to bid farewell to his great-grandfather Louis XIV. Louis advised him not to copy his own mistakes. Do not build so much, do not wage war on your neighbours, and try to improve the lot of ordinary people which he had not. On 1 September 1715 he died. Madame de Maintenon took refuge in the school she had founded at Saint Cyr. Louis was almost 77.

The very next day the Regent removed the infant king and the court from Versailles. It was left empty, and the Duc d'Orléans went straight to the Paris Parlement and persuaded it to overturn the king's will. The bastards were deprived of the young king's education and of their place in the regency council. The Dowager Madame had got her revenge for seeing her royal blood polluted by one of the products of Louis XIV's double adultery with Montespan. The marquise had expired in 1707, very fat. She had not been ordered to leave Versailles by Louis but departed in 1691 because her eldest illegitimate son wanted her apartments, and because she had fallen out with Maintenon, her former employee.

So the regency opened with the child king in the care of the Duc d'Orléans. A very frivolous and fun-loving atmosphere broke out, for a court is dependent upon the character of the centrepiece, and Philippe liked to enjoy life. This allowed Paris to recapture the fashion lead, for George I in London was an old soldier who like his clothes plain and simple. He also subscribed to the Protestant Clothing Ethic that modesty was just as important in a ruler as in his subjects, and that display should be restricted to state occasions. This approach did not exist in France, so the regency glittered.

Elisabeth Charlotte the Dowager Madame survived into 1722, and did not approve of fashionable developments. She wrote on 12 April 1721:

I only follow the fashions from afar, and there are some with which I have nothing to do. Paniers I never wear, and loose gowns [sacques] I abhor and will not even admit into my presence. To me they seem indecent and look as if one has got straight out of bed. There is no method about the fashions here. Tailors, dressmakers, and hairdressers invent them as they please.[17]

She seemed to wish for the system under Louis XIV when fashion was supposed to be launched at court with the king's approval, although how far the mode would obey the monarch was another question. Her easy-going son allowed fashion its head, and was himself so casual as to be portrayed without a cravat and with his shirt wide open. That Louis XIV would never have done, but the reaction against his style was now in full swing. By the end of the year Dowager Madame felt ill and was obliged to wear mantos as a semi-invalid, as they were not boned like the *grand habit*, and could be worn without stays, so they were more comfortable. She even had her manto and petticoats taped together so that she could put them all on together. At 70 in 1722 she closed her eyes. The era of Louis XIV had gone completely and France was no longer in an almost permanent condition of war. The legend began to grow, gilding the events, draping the reign with glory, crowning Versailles with splendour, and the actual cost in thousands of human lives was forgotten. What the people felt about Louis XIV was shown by the dancing in Paris when he died, and the destruction of his statue in the Place Vendôme during the Revolution in 1792. Versailles would be a ruin today, had King Louis Philippe not attended to its restoration in the 1830s.

The styles of Louis XIV's period have been frequently revived. Towering hairstyles began to return to favour from around 1760 but reached proportions that the king would have denounced during the 1770s. The Romantics loved the seventeenth century; the wide collars of Louis XIV's youth appeared again in 1818 and clusters of ringlets over a lady's ears were all the rage in 1835. Prince Albert and Queen Victoria appeared as Louis XIV and Queen Marie Thérèse at one of their fancy-dress balls. Artists from Bonington to Frith liked to recreate scenes of court life in the seventeenth century. The wide sleeves of the 1630s and 1660s were back in fashion in 1830. Occasionally between 1850 and 1860 gowns opened up in front to show the petticoats in the fashion of 1660. In 1869 Worth revived the *cul de crin*, or Baroque bustle, taking 1695/6 as his model, with three tiers of frills on the petticoat. Taller hairstyles returned again, although with greater emphasis on the back of the head as the chief variation. Worth brought bustles back again in 1881 but this time the sweeping trains were reserved for evening dress. Large sleeves came back into vogue over 1890–5, and here too it was in the evening version that they looked most Louis XIV by ending at the elbow. Daytime sleeves reached down to the wrist.

In the twentieth century, a whisper of the revival of bustles was blown away by World War II in 1939. Hoops returned as revived crinolines when Captain Molyneux showed wide skirts in the autumn 1934; by 1937 all Paris was following, and Queen Elizabeth adopted them for the rest of her husband George VI's reign. The bustle effects reappeared in 1983 on Bellville Sassoon's black taffeta and velvet evening gown, and in spring 1984 Ungaro in Paris showed a slim, sugar-rose panné velvet dress with a black lace bow over the backside, falling into a train, which *Vogue* called Baroque use of velvet and lace. Bustle bows and trains were the in thing for bridal gowns by 1986. Louis XIV could have congratulated himself that the styles of his court were still influencing design 300 years later, and Baroque styles, revived so often in the nineteenth and twentieth centuries, have become a major component of Western fashion.

The French cock could also crow over Louis XIV's impact upon court dress. The *grand habit* was adopted by courts across Europe from Spain to Russia, with only Turkey as the exception. Spanish court dress collapsed before it, so that even in Vienna, Madame's grandson's wife the Empress Maria Theresia wore the French *grand habit*; so did her daughters, notably Maria Antonietta, who was thus very familiar with the costume when she went to France to become Marie Antoinette. Although skirts grew much wider, the

bodice, boned with back lacing, cap sleeves, and the double frills or *engageantes* on the shift sleeve, remained constant. For men the embroidered pattern on coats, round the sleevehead, down the seams, down the front of the coat, and down the tails, became established on court uniforms for diplomats, ministers and secretaries of state, so that the style of the *justaucorps* was maintained. In France *justaucorps* persisted until the Revolution in 1789, after which was there no court until Napoleon I crowned himself Emperor. He deliberately tried to create a court dress that was different from his Bourbon predecessors, with no hoops and no bob wigs. As Neo-classical art was the latest ideal, the ladies were now required to dress in classical high waists and white gowns, although trains were allowed to be in coloured velvet. A short puff sleeve discarded the *engageante* frills completely. Nevertheless some seventeenth-century influence persisted, for the men's coats were still embroidered in the same way, although they now had standing collars to decorate. Napoleon also used Baroque ruffs, cravats and plumed hats. His court dress was imposed on his satellite kingdoms of Holland, Spain, Naples and Westphalia. This influenced other courts to imitate, especially the splendid military uniforms, so Austria, Russia, Prussia and Sweden adopted military-style costumes for many court officials in the nineteenth century. The Bourbon restoration of 1814 and 1815, however, saw the Duchesse d'Angoulême, the daughter of Louis XVI, reviving *engageantes* at court, although she teamed them with a high-waisted gown of Empire style. Thus they made a comeback until the collapse of the regime in 1830.

The court of Louis Philippe did not try to impose a court costume, and it became sufficient for ladies to appear in evening dress. Under the Second Napoleonic Empire, ladies had to wear white again, but the dresses could be fashionable. Only the men's coats retained the gold and silver embroidery of Louis XIV's pattern.

Even the British court was influenced by Louis XIV's innovations, although it had a German dynasty from 1714. From 1717 George I began to give receptions at St James's Palace, at Hampton Court and at Windsor Castle.[18] Costume had to be on the French model, the *grand habit de cour* for the ladies, and for the men coats embroidered as on the *justaucorps à brevet* down the seams, around the waist and down the coat tails. Initially the *grand habit* was termed *corps de robe*, but by the 1770s the term *robe de cour* was more usual. The French words reflect the impact of Louis XIV's model.

The skirts of the *grand habit* underwent a major change once round gowns, or closed gowns, began to enter fashion in the 1730s, for they ended the Baroque tradition of exposing the decorated petticoat. As this fashion became established, *grand habits* were given closed skirts, and this variant persisted in France to the Revolution. It was imitated in England, and a description appeared in the *Magazine à la Mode* in January 1777: 'This dress is commonly called a *Robe de Cour*, but more properly the *Royal Robe*, because Her Majesty generally appears in this dress. It consists of a close body, without pleats, or robings, and a train descending from the waist, two and half to three yards long, containing two breadths of silk.'[19]

Ornamentation and trimmings were left to individual fancy, but three tiers of lace ruffles like *engageantes* were compulsory. The men had to wear the French frock, the French version of the British frock coat with narrow cuffs and fur edgings.

While Louis XIV had not laid down any rules over colour for the *grand habit*, and neither did the British court, under Louis XVI in France two changes were made. Debutantes at their first royal presentation had to wear the *grand habit* in black decked with white lace, and on the second day, the *grand habit* in cloth of gold. An alternative to the *grand habit* was introduced by the *Nouvelle Etiquette* of 1773 when the *grande robe à la française* was approved for lesser receptions and ceremonies. It was a revived version of the sacques which Dowager Madame had disapproved of in 1721, when the original loose nature of manto was taken to an extreme by discarding the sash around the waist and increasing the fullness in the back, although the garment remained laced down the front and still covered the shoulders like a normal manto. Such sacque gowns were the rage outside court in the 1720s. Now, 50 years later, a modified version with just two pleats in the back instead of a full flow, allowed the unboned manto to be worn at court instead of the fiercely boned *grand habit*. Thus, exactly a century after its appearance, the manto was elevated to court status. The *grande robe*, as it was now termed, also displayed the petticoat in front, returning to the Baroque tradition, for opening the gown skirt had returned to fashion by 1750. Queen Marie Antoinette changed the ruffles; on the *grand habit* she wore four tiers of frills, instead of the two downwards, two upwards type, and while the *grande robe à la française* retained the cap sleeve of the grand habit, the queen

allowed it to discard *engageantes*, by having only a ruffle at the elbow. The new sacque resembled the grand habit in that both had to be worn with hoops. Fashion had begun to move towards a narrower silhouette, but at court hoops remained.

The British court adopted the *grand habit à la française* and called it for the sake of simplicity 'the sack', although there were only two pleats in the back of the gown. Queen Charlotte adopted the sack and hoop for less grand occasions and continued to wear them long after fashion had moved on.

George III also took inspiration from France in the 1770s when he devised the Windsor uniform for male members of the dynasty. This was a straight copy of the *justaucorps à brevet* in its colouring, for it was in blue with scarlet employed at the collar and cuffs. The uniform was to be worn at Windsor Castle, not elsewhere, so only persons with access to the castle could even be considered for it. The Windsor uniform is still worn for royal birthdays at the castle, so it could be said that one of Louis XIV's innovations is still in use over 300 years later. In Spain the Bourbons introduced the justaucorps for their diplomatic corps, dressing them in dark blue velvet coats, lined with scarlet, and embroidered with silver. Men in fact remained more loyal to the justaucorps than women did to the *grand habit*. Queen Charlotte died in 1818, and George III in 1820, which enabled George IV to abolish the royal robe, the sack and treble ruffles, and the hoop. Henceforth women had only to wear fashionable dress at court, together with trains and ostrich plumes. Embroidered coats for men, however, George IV endorsed, requiring even prime ministers to start to wear uniforms. This met with some opposition. Wellington and Peel were happy to wear Windsor coats at Windsor Castle, but resented having to don a uniform for council meetings with the king, as if they were servants. Attitudes mellowed, however, by the time Victoria reached the throne, for Lord Melbourne wore the civil uniform in black, with gold embroidery across the chest, round the waist and down the tails. The trend towards putting more and more officials into uniform followed Napoleon I's pattern, but the location of the embroidery was a continuation of Louis XIV's *justaucorps à brevet*.

When Louis expired in September 1715, just four days before his 77th birthday, the physician Maréchal ordered the *garçons de la chambre* to change the king's linen, so they probably dressed him in a clean night shirt and nightcap, suitably bedecked with lace. Jean and Jacques Anthoines with the other *garçons* then carried the body to the great parade bed, where it was covered with a pall of cloth of gold. Two altars were set up and as over a hundred priests and monks conducted mass, the courtiers filed past the corpse. The state funeral was on 9 September, setting out in the evening and arriving at St Denis next morning. The *Nouveau Mercure Galant* listed who was at the funeral, then dropped the subject of Louis XIV immediately, and began praising the wisdom, morality and nobility of His Royal Highness the Regent. Power had changed.[20]

His Majesty the King Sun would have had to conclude that women were the most disobedient to his will. Not only did they insist on wearing styles of which he did not approve, but they had even betrayed the success of his *grand habit* in the eighteenth century, by abandoning it for fashionable clothes at court in the nineteenth. Yet his spirit could afford a compensatory smile, for those very fashions do copy the modes of his period, so his impact has endured. Whether it be bustles in 1693, 1779, 1869, 1881 and 1983, or wide collars in 1630–60, 1780, 1819, 1980, there was plenty of attractive shining in the old sun yet. The impact of his court still affects generations after him. If his attempt at glory in his lifetime resulted in Europe uniting against him, over the centuries the glorious legend has persisted. It is a false picture, of course, but one he would not have objected to. The fashions of Versailles will continue to influence design in the years to come. Louis, no doubt, would have said that they should.

Glossary of terms not explained in the text

Carrousel	French equestrian ballet with four quadrilles of riders.
Ell	45 inches.
Galloons	Gold or silver braid, sometimes silk.
Habit de cour	French court dress.
Habit de ville	French fashionable dress, literally town dress.
Lambrequins	French term for classical *pteruges*, the strips into which the sleeves and skirt of Roman military leather tunics were cut to allow easier movement.
Rose of diamonds	A sun-like jewel consisting of a large central diamond surrounded by rays of lesser diamonds.
Undress	Casual attire.

Notes

Introduction: King Sun

1. Athenaïs Pardaillon de Gondrin Marquise de Montespan, *Memoirs*, Nicholl, 1895, p. 77.
2. Françoise Bertaud, Madame de Motteville, *Memoirs*, trs. K. Prescott Wormeley, 1902, vol. I, pp. 105–175; vol. III, p. 44.
3. Anne Marie Louise de Bourbon, Duchesse de Montpensier, *Memoirs of the Grande Mademoiselle 1627–93*, trs. G. Seely, Century Co. New York, 1928, pp. 71–147.
4. Nicolas Sanctot, *Le Sacré de Louis XIV à Reims le 7 Juin 1654*, ed. Abbé Duffo, P. Lethielleux, Paris, 1935, *passim*.
5. John Evelyn, *The Diary*, ed. de Beer, Oxford University Press, 1959.
6. Motteville, op. cit., vol. III, pp. 201–26.
7. Ibid.
8. Andrew Haggard, *Louis XIV in Court and Camp*, Hutchinson, 1904, p. 144.
9. Anne Marie Louise, op. cit., p. 235–43.
10. *Les Pourtraicts de la Cour*, Cologne 1667; English edition, *The Grandeur and Glory of France*, London, 1677, pp. 24-33.
11. François Bluche, 'The Social Origins of the Secretaries of State under Louis XIV', in *Louis XIV and Absolutism*, ed. Ragnhild Hatton, Macmillan, 1976, pp. 85–97.

1 The French Impact 1660–1680

1. Montespan, op. cit. pp. 46–7.
2. Louis de Rouvray, Duc de Saint Simon Vermandois, *Mémoires*, ed. A. de Boislisle, 43 vols. 1879–1930, vol. XXVIII, 'Character of the King'.
3. Marie de Rabutin-Chantal, Marquise de Sevigné, *Letters*, intro. E. Newton, 7 vols, W.T. Morrell, 1928, vol. IV, p. 173.
4. Charles Perrault, *Characters Historical & Panegyrical, of the Greatest Men in France*, trs. J. Ozell, B. Lintott, 1704, p. 206.
5. M. de Marigny, *Les Oeuvres en Vers et en Prose*, Charles de Sercy au Palais, Paris. no date, pp. 35–80.
6. S. Locatelli, *Voyage en France*, pp. 126–206.
7. Montespan, op. cit., p. 10.
8. Marquis de Saint Maurice, *Lettres sur la Cour de Louis XIV 1667–70*, Lemoine Calman-Livry, 1910.
9. Saint Simon, op. cit.
10. Olivier Lefevre d'Ormesson, *Journal 1643–72*, Imprimerie Impériale, Paris, 1861, pp. 405, 552, 577.
11. Charles II, *Letters*, ed. A. Bryant, Cassell, 1935, pp. 89, 225.
12. Sieur de Neuville, *Récit ou Journal du Voiage de M. Claude Lamoral, 11ᵉ Du Nom né le 18 Octobre 1618, Prince du Ligne . . .*, F. Leuridant, 1923, pp. 9, 17, 22–3.
13. Diana de Marly, 'Fashionable Suppliers', *The Antiquaries Journal*, 1979, vol. LVIII pt. 2, pp. 333–51.
14. John Evelyn, *Tyrannus, or The Mode*, 1661, p. 5.
15. Downes, *Roscius Anglicanus*, 1708, p. 29.
16. Anthony Count Hamilton, *Memoirs of Count Gramont*, ed. A. Fea, 1906, p. 188 note 2.
17. Sevigne, op. cit., 4 April 1671.
18. Elisabeth Charlotte Duchesse d'Orléans, *Letters*, ed. G. Scott Stevenson, Chapman & Dodd, 1924, vol. I.
19. Primi Visconti, *Mémoires de la Cour de Louis XIV*, Calman-Levy, *passim*.
20. *Le Mercure Galant*, vol. I, April 1673, p. 86.
21. Sevigné, *Letters*, ed. V. Hammersley, 1955, Secker & Warburg, letter 6.11.76; *Receuil des Lettres de Madame la Marquise de Sevigné à Madame la Comtesse de Grignan*, N. Simart, 1734, vol. IV, pp. 62–3.
22. Montespan, op. cit., p. 158.
23. *Le Nouveau Mercure Galant*, October 1678, pp. 201–9.
24. Sophia Electress of Hanover, *Memoirs*, trs. H. Forrester, Bentley & Son, 1888, pp. 201–45.
25. Marquise de Villars, *Lettres*, Léopold Collin, Paris, 1806, nos. 2, 4.

2 The Textile War

1. Anon., *Life of the Famous John Baptist Colbert*, R. Bentley, 1695, Covent Garden.
2. Maurice Ashley, *Louis XIV and the Greatness of France*, Hodder & Stoughton for English Universities Press, 1949, p. 47.
3. Charles Cole, *Colbert and a Century of French Mercantilism*, Columbia University Press, 1939, vol. I, *passim*.
4. J.B. Colbert, *The Political Testament*, 1695, R. Bentley, Post House, Russell Street, p. 315.
5. Cole, op. cit., vol. II, pp. 136, 150, 207, 246; Diana de Marly 'Pepys and the Fashion for Collecting', *Costume*, no. 21, 1987.
   Gobelin was founded in 1440 by the scarlet dyer Jean Gobelin. It still exists at 42 Avenue des Gobelins, near the Porte d'Italie, Paris.
6. E. Pariset, *Histoire de la Fabrique Lyonnaise*, A. Rey, Lyons, 1901, pp. 90–3.
7. *Statutes at Large, Charles II*, ed. Danby Pickering, Cambridge, 1763, pp. 228, 240, 440.
8. *Calendar of State Papers, Domestic Series*, 1660–70, ed. Mary Anne Everett Green, 1860, vol. 1665–6, p. 31.
9. *CSPD supra*, 1670, p. 601.
10. *CSPD*, ed. F. Blackburne Daniell, 1895, vol. 1673–5, pp. 315–6.
11. *CSPD*, 1676–77, pp. 18–19, Secretary Williamson's notes at the Committee of Trade.
12. *CSPD*, 1672–3, pp. 288, 304.
13. *CSPD*, March 1675–Feb. 1676, p. 211.
14. *CSPD*, William & Mary, 1690–5.
15. Pierre Gaxotte, *La France de Louis XIV*, Hachette, Paris 1946, pp. 239–54.
16. *The Quiet Conquest*, catalogue of the Huguenot exhibition, Museum of London, 1985, pp. 289–306, 'Huguenots in the Silk Industry'.
17. Ibid., p. viii, cat. nos. 269, 270, 262.
18. Diderot and d'Alembert, *Encyclopédie ou Dictionnaire Raisonné des Sciences Arts, et des Métiers*, Samuel Fauluche, Neufchastel, 1765.
19. *The Works of M. Boileau*, E. Sayer at the Post House, E. Curll at the Dial & Bible Fleet Street, 1712.
20. John Haynes, *A View of the Present State of the Clothing Trade in England with Remarks of the Causes and Pernicious Consequences of its Decay*, 1706, pp. 10–36.
21. Louis XIV, *East India Goods*, 1686.

3 Court Dress and Masquerades

1. Information from Madame M. Delpierre, Museé de la Mode, Paris.
2. Marquis de Sourches, *Mémoires sur la Règne de Louis XIV*, ed. le Comte de Cosnac & E. Pontal, 13 vols, Hachette, Paris 1883, vol. II, Feb. 1688, vol. III, 22 Sept. 1691.
3. Pierre Larousse, *Grande Dictionnaire Universel de XIXe Siècle*, Paris, 1873.
4. *The Letters of Madame*, trs. & ed. Gertrude Scott Stevenson, Chapman & Dodd, 1924, vol. I, p. 116.
5. Saint Simon. op. cit.
6. Montespan, op. cit., vol. II, p. 93.
7. Madame La Mothe, Comtesse d'Aulnoy, *Memoirs of the Court of Spain*, trs. T. Brown, 1692, Part I, pp. 61–2, Part II, pp. 49, 85–6.
8. Ruth Matilda Anderson, 'The Golilla, A Spanish Collar of the 17th Century', *Waffen und Kostumkunde*, Munich, 1969–70, pp. 1–19.
9. Malcolm Rogers, *William Dobson 1611–46*, catalogue of National Portrait Gallery exhibition 1938–4, plates 17, 18, colour plates 5, 7, and plate 31.
10. B. Naderzad, 'Louis XIV, La Boullaye et l'Exotisme Persan', *Gazette des Beaux Arts*, vol. 71, 1972, pp. 29–38.
11. C.F. Menestrier, *Traité des Tournois, Ioustes, Carrousels et autres spectacles publics*, Lyons, 1669, pp. 198–203.
12. Lord Chamberlain Warrants, LC 7/1, 12 July 1661, Public Record Office.
13. Madame La Mothe, Comtesse d'Aulnoy, *Memoirs of the Court of England*, English edition 1707, pp. 485–95.
14. Abbé de Choisy, *Mémoires pour servir à l'histoire de Louis XIV*; Wan-de-Vater, Utrecht, 1727, p. 153.
15. Brian Bevan, *Charles II's Minette*, Ascent Books, 1979, pp. 61, 77, 135.
16. Madame de la Fayette, *Memoirs of the Court of France for the Years 1688–9*, Routledge, 1929, p. 199.
17. *12th Report of Commission on Historical Manuscripts, Manuscripts of the Duke of Rutland at Belvoir Castle*, Appendix V, 1889, letters 1685/6.
18. Hamilton, op. cit., pp. 131–9.
19. Sigrid Flamand Christensen, *Kongedragterne fra 17 og 18 Aarhundrede*, Copenhagen, 1940, cat. nos. 57–68.
20. *Le Nouvelle Mercure Galant*, the Palace, Paris, February 1679, pp. 150–85. For the tailor Baraillon see Diana de Marly, *Costume on the Stage*, Batsford, 1982, p. 28.
21. Philippe de Courcillon, Marquis de Dangeau, *Memoirs of the Court of France*, trs. John Davenport, Henry Collins, 1825, entries for 18 Feb. 1685–Jan 1686.

4 Fashion 1680–1700

1. Visconti, op. cit., pp. 267, p. 304.
2. Montespan, op. cit., II, pp. 93–5.
3. Ibid.
4. Georges Durand, 'What is Absolutism?', in *Louis XIV and Absolutism*, op. cit., pp. 18–38.
5. Visconti, op. cit., p. 136.
6. *Receuil des Lettres de Mme de Sevigné*, IV, pp. 418–19.
7. Maria Kroll, *Sophia Electress of Hanover*, Victor Gollancz, 1973, pp. 159–62.
8. Sourches, op. cit., I, pp. 9–10.

9. Saint Simon, op. cit.

10. Veronika Gervers, *The Influence of Ottoman Turkish Textiles and Costume in Eastern Europe*, Royal Ontario Museum, 1982, p. 12: Thokoly owned 16 Turkish kaftans in the 1683–6 inventory. Dangeau, op. cit., 27 January 1687. In the West robes were given as part of livery, as in the Byzantine Empire in the tenth century: one ceremonial robe to patricians per annum, two robes to magistrates; admirals and similar ranks four robes: *vide* George Ostrogorsky, *History of the Byzantine State*, 1984, p. 252 n. 2.

11. Blenheim Palace, Ms.E.19.

12. *Letters from Liselotte*, trs. ed. Maria Kroll, letter of 10 June 1687.

13. Mary Evelyn, *Mundus Muliebris, or The Ladies Dressing-Room Unlock'd*, 1690, intro. J. Nevinson, reprint by Costume Society, 1977.

14. *Letters of Madame*, op. cit., I, p. 78.

15. Maria Kroll, op. cit., pp. 179, 200.

16. Lucy Norton, *First Lady of Versailles*, Hamish Hamilton, 1978, p. 21.

17. *Le Nouveau Mercure Galant*, December 1697, pp. 206–60; and August 1698, pp. 234–41.

18. *Le Nouveau Mercure Galant*, October 1698, pp. 258–87.

19. *Gazette d'Amsterdam*, no. LXXXI 2 and 9 October 1699.

5 Conclusion 1700–1715

1. Lionel Kochan, *The Making of Modern Russia*, Cape, 1962, p. 111.

2. *Le Nouveau Mercure Galant*, Feb. 1700, pp. 155–233.

3. *Letters from Liselotte*, op. cit., *Secret Memoirs*, 19 Feb. 1702.

4. Elisabeth Charlotte, *Secret Memoirs*, p. 53.

5. Collection Society of Antiquaries of London, broadside no. 619.

6. Ruth Jordan, *Sophia Dorothea 1666–1726*, Constable, 1971, pp. 153, 214.

7. *Letters from Liselotte*, op. cit., 26 June 1701.

8. Ibid., 25 Feb. 1706.

9. *Le Nouveau Mercure Galant*, Nov. 1708, p. 150.

10. Saint Simon, Vol. XXI, 1910, pp. 35–6.

11. Anon., *The Present State of the Court of France*, 1712, pp. 16–49.

12. Maria Kroll, op. cit., pp. 222–3.

13. *The Letters of Madame*, op. cit., I, p. 272.

14. Saint Simon, XXIII, 1911, pp. 284–6; Diana de Marly, 'The Vocabulary of the Female Headdress', *Waffen und Kostumkunde*, 1975, part 1, pp. 61–70.

15. *Letters from Liselotte*, 1 Oct. 1712.

16. Saint Simon, XVIII, 1891, pp. 33; XXVIII, 1916, p. 40.

17. *Letters of Madame*, op. cit., II, p. 267.

18. John Beattie, *The English Court in the Reign of George I*, Cambridge, 1967, *passim*.

19. *Magazine à la Mode, or Fashionable Miscellany*, J. Wenman, Fleet Street, Jan. 1777, p. 4.

20. Jean and Jacques Anthoines, *La Mort de Louis XIV*, Quantin, Paris, 1880, pp. 75, 80.

Money

The French livre was worth 20 sols, or shillings, and was the equivalent of a pound sterling, but its value declined greatly. There were several types of livre in France; according to Randle Cotgrave's *Dictionary of the French and English Tongues* 1611 the values were:

livre Barrois: 14 sols *c.* 18d.
livre Bourdelois: 12½ sols, worth half a Paris pound.
livre Mansais: 4/−.
livre Parisis: 7 sols, or 2/6.

livre Tournois: 10 to the English pound, 2/−.
Ecu or Escu: the French crown, or 5/−.
Pistole: Spanish gold coin worth between 16/6 and 18/−.
The livre Tournois was the most common and in 1670 was worth about 1/4.
The franc was worth sols Tournois 20, or 2/−.
franc Bourdelois: 18d.
franc à cheval: an old gold coin, now worth 2/−.
franc à pied: 4 to 5/−.
Louis d'or: gold coin worth 25 francs.

The Royal Wardrobe

The wardrobe was a sub-department of the grand chamberlain's office. It consisted of two masters of the wardrobe, four first valets, 16 ordinary valets, and three tailors-breechmakers (*tailleurs-chaussetiers*). In 1669 the master was the Marquis of Guitry, and in 1670 the Marquis of Soyecourt. The valets served for the quarter year under the following system:

First valets		Valets
Jan.	M. Rose	Lissolde, Belot, Ronquerolles, d'Orval.
April	M. Moreau	Limonet, and son, Gûle, Richcome, l'Abbé.
July	M. Guitonneau	de Courbaçon, and son, l'Escluse, Herbergeon, Rossignol.
Oct.	M. Talon	de la Fosse, Brice, Chaillot, Barrois.
Tailors:	Ourdault and nephew.	
	de S. Germain.	
	Etienne Taburet and son.	

The tailors also had the rank of valets of the bedchamber which enabled them to assist in dressing the king. When the king awoke, the valet of the bedchamber on duty took him his nightgown (dressing gown). The first valet of the wardrobe then delivered the understockings, and placed the left stocking on the king's left leg. The first valet of the bedchamber put the right understocking on the right leg. Another valet of the wardrobe brought the silk stockings which were attached to the drawers, and the king usually put these on himself. The pages of the bedchamber then brought the king's mules or slippers. A valet of the wardrobe then delivered the kneebreeches, and the shoes which he knotted. If the king decided to wear boots the spurs had to be attached by the master of the horse or his equerry. The valets of the wardrobe then brought the king's shirt, to hand to the master of the wardrobe, the grand chamberlain, or the first gentleman of the bedchamber, who all had the right of presenting the shirt to the king, unless a prince of the blood were present in which case he performed the duty. The master of the wardrobe then helped the king into his doublet, cloak, cravat, and presented the gloves, handkerchief, and sword. A similar performance was conducted when the king retired for the night.

The queen also had an establishment with a master of the wardrobe, first valets, and valets, but her staff served for half the year, not the quarter year which the king's staff served. In addition she had four *tapissiers* to look after the tapestry and upholstery, who served as follows: January to July: Le Roux, P. Noroy; July to December: N. Noroy, P. Miche. The Queen employed four embroiderers of whom only two were named: Guillot and Le Clerc. Her tailors, four in number, also served half-yearly: January to July: Iossant called Le Clos, and Richard called Le Comte; July to December: Classe and Garnier.

The household of the king's brother Monsieur Philippe Duc d'Orléans had a similar system with a master of the wardrobe, four first valets and 12 valets. One of his tailors was the same as the king's Taburet and son, and his other was François Seriny. The lady's tailor to the duchesse, Henriette Anne, was Jean Quan, and to her daughters Marie Louise and Anne Marie, François Laye.

Costumes for carrousels, operas, ballets, masques, masquerades and similar extraordinaries were designed by the Cabinet du Roi, where the chief designers were Henri Gissey, 1621–73, and Jean Berain the elder, 1637–1711. The designs were made up by the tailor Jean Baraillon who must have been the largest entertainments' costumier in Paris, as he made clothes for the King's Ballet, the Comédie Française, the Théatre du Palais Royal, the Théatre de Guénégaud in addition to dressing the king's *divertissements*. The orders for the king's clothes were the duty of the first gentlemen of the bedchamber.

The Crown employed another 26 tailors outside the wardrobe and Cabinet, whose names were not listed, plus 8 perfumed glovemakers of whom Martial was the most famous, 14 shoe and bootmakers, 8 embroiderers, 4 sashmakers, and 2 silk and woollen stocking makers. The permission in 1675 for women to be professional dressmakers resulted in Madame Lebrion instead of a male tailor being appointed *couturière* to the Duchesse de Bourgogne. Her firm was in the rue de la Vieille Monnaie, in which area could be found other dressmakers such as Mesdames Charpentier and de Villeneuve. The king's silkmercer Charlier was in the rue de la Couttellerie. The chief woollen draper was Gaultier. The royal barber in 1669 was Prud'homme, who was later succeeded by Quentin. There were also eight barbers on call who worked on the quarter system. Quentin supplied some of the king's periwigs, and so did Evrais. Madame Quentin was maid and briefly mistress of the robes to the Duchesse de Bourgogne. Cravats came from M. de Miramond. The embroiderers l'Herminot and the brothers Delobel were accommodated at Versailles, on easy call for sewing crown jewels on to clothes. The most fashionable ladies' hair stylists were Madame de Sénécé in the 1640s, and Madame Martin in the 1670s. The shoemaker responsible for Monsieur's high heels was Lambertin.

Chief sources:
L'Etat de France, Jean Guignard, 1669, Vol. I., *passim.*
Le Nouveau Mercure Galant 1677–1679.

Bibliography

ANON., *L'Etat de France*, Jean Guignard, 1669, Paris.
Life of John Baptiste Colbert, R. Bentley, 1695.
Les Pourtraicts de la Cour, Cologne, 1667.
The Present State of the Court of France, and City of Paris, in a Letter from Monsieur M. to the Honourable Matthew Prior Esq., one of the Commissioners of Her Majesty's Customs, E. Curl, 1712.

ANDERSON, Ruth, 'The Golilla, A Spanish Collar of the 17th Century', *Waffen und Kostumkunde*, Munich, 1969–70, pp. 1–19.

ANTHOINES, Jean and Jacques, *La mort de Louis XIV*, Quantin, Paris, 1880.

ASHLEY, Maurice, *Louis XIV and the Greatness of France*, Hodder & Stoughton for the English Universities Press, 1949.

BEATTIE, John, *The English Court in the Reign of George I*, Cambridge, 1967.

BEVAN, Brian, *Charles II's Minette*, Ascent Books, 1979.

BLUCHE, François, 'The Social Origins of the Secretaries of State under Louis XIV', in *Louis XIV and Absolutism*, ed. Ragnhild Hatton, Macmillan, 1976.

BOILEAU, *The Works*, E. Sayer at the Post House, E. Curll at the Dial & Bible Fleet Street, 1712.

Calendar of State Papers, Domestic Series, ed. Mary Everett Green to 1670 and F.H. Blackburne Daniell thereafter, Longman, Brown, Green, Longman & Roberts, 1858–1904.

CHARLES II, *Letters*, ed. A. Bryant, Cassell, 1935.

CHRISTENSEN, Sigrid Flamand, *Kongedragterne fra 17 og 18 Aarhundrede*, Copenhagen, 1940.

COLBERT, Jean Baptiste, *The Political Testament*, R. Bentley, Post House, Russell Street, 1695.

COLE, Charles, *Colbert and a Century of French Mercantilism*, Columbia University Press, 1939.

Commission on Historical Manuscripts, 12th Report, Manuscripts of the Duke of Rutland at Belvoir Castle, 1889.

COWPER, Mary, Countess, *Diary 1714–20*, John Murray, 1864.

D'AULNOY, Madame La Mothe, Comtesse, *Memoirs of the Court of England*, 1707.
Memoirs of the Court of Spain, T. Brown, 1692.

DE BOURBON, Anne Marie Louise, Duchesse de Montpensier, *Memoirs of the Grande Mademoiselle*, 1627–93, trs. G. Seely, Century Co., New York, 1928.

DE CHOISY, Abbé, *Memoires pour servir à l'histoire de Louis XIV*, Wan-de-Vater, Utrecht, 1727.

DE COURÇILLON, Philippe, Marquis de Dangeau, *Memoirs of the Court of France*, trs. John Davenport, Henry Collin, 1825.

DE GONDRIN Athenaïs Pardaillon, Marquise de Montespan, *Memoirs*, Nichols, 1895.

DE LA FAYETTE, Madame, *Memoirs of the Court of France for the Years 1688–9*, Routledge, 1929.

DE LIONNE, Hugues, *Lettres Inédites*, Chenevier, Valence, 1877.

DE MARLY, Diana, 'Fashionable Suppliers, Leading Tailors and Clothing Tradesmen of the Restoration Period', *The Antiquaries Journal*, 1979, vol. LVIII, part 2.
Costume on the Stage 1600–1940, Batsford, 1982.

DE MOTTEVILLE, Françoise Bertaud, Madame, *Memoirs*, trs. K. Prescott Wormeley, W. Heinemann, 1902.

DE LA NEUVILLE, *Récit ou Journal de Voiage de M. Claude Lamoral, 11ᵉ Du Nom né le 18 Octobre 1618, Prince de Ligne, du Sainte Empire et D'Amblise, par son ambassade de S.M.C. vers le Roy de la Grande Bretagne à l'an 1660*, Felicient Leuridant, Brussels, 1923.

DE RABUTIN-CHANTAL, Marie, Marquise de Sevigné, *Receuil des Lettres de Madame la Marquise de Sevigné à Madame la Comtesse de Grignan*, N. Simart, Paris, 1734.
Letters, intro. E. Newton, W.T. Morrell, 1928.
Letters, ed. V. Hammersley, Secker & Warburg, 1955.

DE ROUVRAY, Louis Duc de Saint Simon Vermandois, *Mémoires*, ed. A. de Boislisle, 43 vols, 1879–1930.

DE SAINT MAURICE, Marquis, *Lettres sur la Cour de Louis XIV 1667–70*, Lemoine Calman-Livry, 1910.

DE SOURCHES, Marquis, *Mémoires sur la Règne de Louis XIV*, ed le Comte de Cosnac & E Pontal, 13 vols, Hachette, Paris, 1883.

DE VILLARS, Marquise, *Letters*, Léopold Collin, Paris, 1806.

DIDEROT & D'ALEMBERT, *Encyclopédie, or Dictionnaire Raisonné des Sciences, Arts et Métiers*, S. Faluche, Neufchastel, 1765.

D'ORMESSON, Olivier Lefevre, *Journal 1643–72*, Imprimerie Impériale, Paris, 1861.

DOWNES, John, *Roscius Anglicanus*, 1708.

DURAND, Georges, 'What is Absolutism?' in *Louis XIV and Absolutism*, ed. Ragnhild Hatton, Macmillan, 1976.

EVELYN, John, *Tyrannus, or, The Mode*, 1661.
The Diary, ed. de Beer, Oxford University Press, 1959.

EVELYN, Mary, *Mundus Muliebris; or, The Ladies Dressing-Room Unlock'd*, 1690, intro. J. Nevinson, Costume Society reprint, 1977.

GAXOTTE, Pierre, *La France de Louis XIV*, Hachette, 1946.
Gazette d'Amsterdam.
Gazette de France.
Gervers, Veronika, *The Influence of Ottoman Turkish Textiles and Costume in Eastern Europe*, Royal Ontario Museum, 1982.

HAGGARD, Andrew, *Louis XIV in Court and Camp*, Hutchinson, 1904.

HAMILTON, Anthony, Count, *Memoirs of Count Gramont*, ed. Allan Fea, Bickers & Son, 1906.

HATTON, Ragnhild, *Louis XIV and Europe*, Macmillan, 1976.

HAYNES, John, *A View of the Present State of the Clothing Trade in England with Remarks on the Causes and Pernicious Consequences of its Decay*, 1706.

JORDAN, Ruth, *Sophia Dorothea, 1666–1726*, Constable, 1971.

KOCHAN, Lionel, *The Making of Modern Russia*, Cape, 1962.

KROLL, Maria, *Sophia Electress of Hanover*, Victor Gollancz, 1973.

LAROUSSE, Pierre, *Grande Dictionnaire Universel du XIXe Siècle*, Larousse, Paris, 1873.

LOCATELLI, Sebastiano, *Voyage en France*, A. Vautier, Paris, 1905.

LOUIS XIV, *Mémoires de Louis XIV pour L'Instruction du Dauphin*, ed. Charles Dreyss, Didier, Paris, 1860.
Declaration du Roy par laquelle sa Maiesté en interpretant celle du 27 Novembre 1660 permet à tous ses Sujets de porter des passemens et dentelles de fil et de soye, du prix et de la façon mentionnez en la presente Declaration, 30 Juin 1661.
Declaration du Roy portant deffences de porter des Etoffes et Passemens d'or et d'argent, ny mesme des dentelles de fil des pays Estrangers, 23 Nov. 1667. This repeated restrictions of 1660, 1661 and 1664.
Arrest du Conseil d'Estat, 17 Mars 1668 portant iteratives deffences de vendre, porter, debiter aucuns points Estrangers, tant que commencez d'user.

Regelemens des manufactures de draps d'or, d'argent et de soye, établi en la Ville, Faubourgs et Ban-lieue de Paris, et le reglemen général de toutes sortes de teintures de Soye, Laines Fils, qui s'employent aus dites Manufactures, Tapisseries et autres Etoffes et Ouvrages, 13 Aout 1669.
East India Goods 26 Oct. 1686.

Magazine à la Mode, or Fashionable Miscellany, J. Wenman, Fleet Street, 1777.

MARIGNY, M., *Les Oeuvres en Vers et en Prose*, Charles de Sercy au Palais, Paris, no date.

MENESTRIER, C.F., *Traité de Tournois, Ioustes, Carrousels, et autres Spectacles Publics*, Lyons, 1669.

Le Mercure Galant, 1672–3, Paris.

The Mercury Galant, trs. John Dancer, 1673, London.

Museum of London, *The Quiet Conquest*, 1985.

NADERZAD, B. 'Louis XIV, La Boullaye et l'Exotisme Persan', *Gazette des Beaux Arts*, 1972.

NORTON, Lucy, *First Lady of Versailles*, Hamish Hamilton, 1978.

Le Nouveau Mercure Galant, from 1677.

ORLEANS, Elisabeth Charlotte Duchesse d', and Dowager Duchess from 1701, *Secret Memoirs of the Court of Louis XIV*, Grohier Society, 1904.
The Letters of Madame, trs. & ed. Gertrude Scott Stevenson, Chapman and Dodd, 1924.
The Letters of Liselotte, trs. & ed. Maria Kroll, Gollancz, 1970. (Liselotte was Madame's German pet name)

PARISET, E. *Histoire de la Fabrique Lyonnaise*, A. Rey, Lyons, 1901.

PERRAULT, Charles, *Characters Historical and Panegyrical of the Greatest Men of France*, trs. J. Ozell, B. Lintott, 1704.

PRIOR, Matthew, *Memoirs of the Life of Matthew Prior*, E. Curll at the Dial & Bible, 1722.

SANCTOT, Nicolas, *Le Sacré de Louis XIV à Reims, 7 Juin 1654*, ed. Abbé Duffo, P. Lethielleux, Paris, 1935.

SOPHIA OF HANOVER, *Memoirs, 1630–80*, trs. H. Forester, Bentley & Son, 1888.

VISCONTI, Primi, Jean Baptiste, Comte de Saint Mayol, *Mémoires sur la Cour de Louis XIV*, trs. into French from Italian by Jean Lemoine, Calman-Lévy, Paris, 1908.

Manuscripts

Lord Chamberlain's Warrants, LC 7/1, 1661, Public Record Office.

Blenheim Palace Ms.E.19. coll. the Duke of Marlborough.

Index